KT-364-092

A User's Guide to the Penis

Members Club

PIET HOEBEKE

GREEN TREE
LONDON · OXFORD · NEW YORK · NEW DELHI · SYDNEY

GREEN TREE
Bloomsbury Publishing Plc
50 Bedford Square, London, WC1B 3DP, UK

BLOOMSBURY, GREEN TREE and the Green Tree logo are trademarks
of Bloomsbury Publishing Plc

First published in Great Britain, 2020

Translated by Tanya Behiels

A catalogue record for this book is available from the British Library

Library of Congress Cataloguing-in-Publication data has been applied for

ISBN: HB: 978-1-4729-7760-1; eBook: 978-1-4729-7759-5; ePDF: 978-1-4729-7758-8

2 4 6 8 10 9 7 5 3 1

Typeset in Dante MT by Deanta Global Publishing Services, Chennai, India
Printed and bound in Great Britain by CPI Group (UK) Ltd, Croydon CR0 4YY

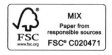

To find out more about our authors and books visit www.bloomsbury.com
and sign up for our newsletters

I dedicate this book to all my patients who have a penis that differs from the norm, but who live a life close to perfection.

You prove each and every day that it doesn't matter what kind of penis you have. The most important thing is how you live with it.

I admire you for that.

Contents

Introduction

When I was younger, I actually wanted to be a vet. As a child, I dreamed of helping sick animals, but in the end I chose to train as a doctor. I found animals didn't have much to say.

During my first few years as a medical student, I never could have guessed that I would specialise in the urinary tract and genitalia. A body has so many fascinating organs and structures – the penis didn't immediately stand out as the most interesting part. I knew I wanted to operate on people and that I wanted to be more than your average surgeon. Many surgeons work on behalf of a specialist and don't see the patients again after the surgery. An abdominal surgeon, for example, will often do a lot of treatment for diagnoses already made by the specialist gastroenterologist, and then not be involved with the patient again. That didn't appeal to me. I wanted to diagnose patients and then support them throughout their treatment, from start to finish.

Wanting to do something both surgical and diagnostic left me with relatively few options – you either became a urologist (working on genitalia) or an otorhinolaryngologist (working on mouth, nose and ears). Urology fitted best with my ambitions. It was a wide-reaching field; it not only covered the penis, but also the kidneys and bladder. It even covered cancer.

Armed with much enthusiasm, but no definite career plan, I became a urologist in training at Ghent University Hospital. I followed my interests and by all kinds of chance occurrences, new worlds opened up to me.

In autumn 1992, the urology department at the hospital was going through a difficult time. I was still in training, but had operated on, or assisted in operations of, barely two hundred patients or so in a year. I felt I had far too little experience to become a specialist urologist, as the Programme Committee required. The then dean and chief physician at the University Hospital knew I was concerned. They advised me to do a year abroad. 'By the time you come back, we'll have sorted things out and you can continue your training position here,' they promised.

I went to the Wilhelmina Children's Hospital in Utrecht in the Netherlands and there I met a remarkable colleague in the paediatric urology department, Tom de Jong. He introduced me to the fascinating world of congenital disorders of the urinary tract and sex organs. This is what I specialised in.

This is how, quite unexpectedly, I performed my first operation on a trans woman.

A year later, when I returned to Ghent, the dean and chief physician had kept their word – a new department head, Wim Oosterlinck, had taken over the running of the department and things were far better organised. Wim immediately asked me to put paediatric urology on the map in Belgium.

A new wave of serendipity sent me in the direction of transgender patients – people who feel like a man in the body of a woman, or vice versa. Or, from a urologist's perspective, people who don't have a penis but want one, or vice versa.

Professor Guido Matton, a famous name in plastic surgery, was the first to perform the operation to turn a penis into a clitoris in a trans woman in Ghent in 1987. As chance would have it, I was on call, assisting in a prostate resection in a nearby theatre. I was suddenly called to help Professor Matton, who couldn't find the nerve leading to the tip of the penis. I showed the professor what he was looking for and he wouldn't let me leave. This is how, quite unexpectedly, I performed my first operation on a trans woman. Afterwards, the Professor said to me, 'Right, from now on, you can help me anytime.'

I did transgender surgery from then on, and I've been doing it for 25 years. For the first few years, I operated on trans women, but from 1996 onwards, my patients were mainly trans men – biological women who wanted a male body.

Five years ago, I stopped doing these operations. Something had been bothering me about them for a while. Instead of sleeping, I would lie in bed worrying and didn't know why. During a holiday in Israel with my husband Roberto and our two best friends, overlooking the incredible view of the river valley in Be'er Sheva, we chatted about my sleeplessness and my work. Suddenly, the pieces of the puzzle fitted together.

I treated trans people with heart and soul, but I was weighed down by the number of patients there were and, in particular, the complications which some of them were fighting with. I was a *second victim*, I realised. That is a typical phenomenon for doctors. It starts with trouble sleeping, and if you don't do anything about it, you start to get nightmares, lose your self-confidence and are overcome by severe startle responses. The next stage is burnout.

It was then that I knew I could no longer handle the complications. The patients coming to me were getting younger and younger, and the complications more and more painful. I made a decision: I would stop operating on trans people.

I stuck to that decision for a few years, until I felt I was free from my 'second victim' problem. I have since started treating trans men again, albeit less than before and always together with two colleagues. That takes the pressure off my shoulders.

However, I continued to operate on biological men who, for one reason or another, were born without a penis or who had lost their penis in an accident. For these patients, we make a new penis, and that entails fewer complications than the genital reconstruction required in trans people.

There is also another kind of procedure that I'm doing less and less, but for a very different reason than my psychological burden. In the course of my career, opinions have changed about some procedures and therefore so has the way in which I go about them. I'm talking about children with both male and female sexual characteristics.

During my year in the Netherlands, I was not only fascinated by paediatric urology, but also by differences in sex development – something we used to call 'intersexuality'. This involves differences in the three levels of sex that someone has. First, there is genetic sex – your DNA says whether you are a male or female. Then, there is gonadal sex – you have testicles or ovaries. Finally, there is external sex – a penis or vulva. The three levels of sex are usually the same in most people, but they can also vary in some people.

For example, someone can have the typical XY chromosomes of a man but look like a woman on the outside, i.e. with a vulva instead of a penis – and with testicles in her abdomen. There are hundreds of variations that deviate from the traditional 'difference' between man and woman. Just thinking about the way in which such deviations occur, and why, was something that always kept me busy.

When I moved back to Ghent from Utrecht, I immediately set up a special group of colleagues to consider the diagnosis and treatment of such conditions. We were the first – and, as yet, still the only – multidisciplinary centre in Belgium fundamentally dealing with children with differences in sex development, and their parents. Simply put, we were dealing with boys who were not developing sufficiently as males or girls who were developing with male characteristics.

Treatment was simple: boys who weren't male enough underwent surgery to strengthen their male characteristics, girls underwent surgery to strengthen their female characteristics.

I use the past tense very consciously here. Our surgical model was heavily based on the dichotomy between male and female: you were either one or the other and, as a child, it was best to be placed in the right category as soon as possible, if necessary with the help of surgery. This strict categorisation didn't stand the test of time. There is no longer a wall standing between male and female. We discovered that it is more like a spectrum, a gradual transition. Gender fluidity has become more widespread than the traditional division of male and female, and it is therefore no longer taken for granted that young children should be operated on without them first giving their consent. Just because mummy and daddy want a 'normal' girl or 'normal' boy, it doesn't mean that child should be moulded to their wishes. You never know how such a child will develop, and that is why we now prefer to wait.

My entire professional career pivots around the three core areas that crossed my path by chance: congenital urological and genital disorders, transsexuality and differences in sex development. I saw penises of all shapes and sizes. Some people only felt complete once they finally had a penis between their legs. Others couldn't get rid of theirs quickly enough. Many patients feel miserable because they think their perfectly normal penis is too small. Others feel like the king of the world when their clitoris becomes a micropenis.

The best part isn't when an operation has been successful, but when someone feels you have really helped them. I therefore still love my work.

What continues to interest me is the relationship between the body and how people experience sexuality. For men, there is no escaping the penis. No, men don't think with their penis, but the penis is an extension of the brain more than any other organ. That's not just because of the many neural pathways between the penis and the brain, but also because of the psychology of sexuality and the libido, which all goes on in the brain.

Some find penises nice to look at, others find them ugly. But what always stands true is that the identification of a man is largely related to his penis. Even if they have a perfectly normal specimen, men still worry about it. Is it stiff enough? Does it ejaculate enough sperm? Does it turn women off?

Approximately half the world's population has a penis, and the other half regularly make use of one. Some people have a penis and don't want one, others don't have a penis and do want one. Some men get rid of their penis, others think theirs is too small, too bent, too limp or too thin. In very rare cases, they complain that their penis is too long or too wide. Sometimes a penis has an abnormality and we need to operate, other penises are circumcised without any medical need.

Wherever there are people, there are penises, but even though penises exist all over the world, a lot of ignorance still surrounds them.

Wherever there are people, there are penises, but even though penises exist all over the world, a lot of ignorance still surrounds them. There are so many myths out there, which means that useful knowledge often doesn't get through. All these myths burden men with frustrations, and I unfortunately have met too many men – young and old – whose quality of life completely diminished because they had a false image of their penis.

What is the penis and why is it what it is? How should you look after that sausage-shaped organ and can you 'train' your penis?

Nearly every man is born with one, but it doesn't come with a user manual. Let's do something about that with this book.

1

And then came the penis

Why do men have a penis?

All men – correction – *nearly* all men, have a penis. But why?

Our distant ancestors didn't have penises at all. When a man met a woman and they wanted to make babies, she laid eggs and he discharged his milt (semen) over them. That wasn't easy, because they lived in water. Our (very) distant ancestors were fish after all and most types of fish still don't have a penis.

One blue moon, some fish had had enough of all that water and they crawled ashore. From those pioneers came amphibians. Amphibians still need water to breed, which explains why frogs don't have a penis either.

When you can only reproduce with enough water nearby, you're not, unfortunately, free to roam the world. So reptiles invented internal fertilisation – the females mimicked the wet conditions of the frog pond inside their bodies. This meant they could be fertilised wherever they wanted, even without any water in sight. All that was needed was for the male to have an organ that would bring his sperm into contact with the eggs inside the female's body.

And thus the penis took to the stage. We are still walking around with that organ today.

As with all other mammals, fertilisation takes place internally in humans and the penis is the instrument with which the sperm cells are delivered to the female partner. Once an egg is fertilised, it grows into a foetus in the womb. Without internal fertilisation, men wouldn't have a penis and we would only be able to reproduce by cuddling up in a bath or pond. At least the penis doesn't stop us from still enjoying a nice warm bubble bath! Birds, the descendants of dinosaurs, have since lost their penis. Only 3 per cent of bird species still have one. In all other species, the male has to press his cloaca (opening for stool, urine and sperm) against the female's to sow his seed. If humans had gone down that route, too, we wouldn't have gynaecologists and urologists today, only cloacologists.

The penis initially came about for reproduction, but the chance events of evolution found a sideline for it: it is also used as the body's drainage channel. Ejaculation and urination take place via the same tract, even though sperm and urine have very different biological functions: the purpose of sperm is to find a fertile place, while urine removes waste substances from the body.

For young boys, their penis is mainly a tool for urinating, an attachment for which there is no other conceivable purpose. Only in puberty do they discover that urinating is only one thing you can use a penis for. It is then that they begin to understand why girls don't have one, even though they still urinate.

With the penis serving as a drainage channel, men make good use of it to urinate standing up. However, when you look at the internal plumbing system, you soon see that urinating while standing isn't the intention at all. I'll come back to this later.

Major transformations

You don't just get a penis because you have male genes. Before birth, foetuses have to work hard to become a male – if they don't, they stay female.

Have no illusions: in the womb, we are all the same to begin with. At the very beginning, there are no differences between male and female genitalia. Both the clitoris and the penis develop from the same structure, the primordial phallus. Then there are the labioscrotal swellings, which either develop into a scrotum or into labia. Every embryo can potentially develop into a human with male or female sex organs.

The difference lies in the chromosomes. Every human has 46 chromosomes, divided into pairs. In a female, the 23rd pair consists of two X chromosomes. A male only **Both the clitoris and the penis develop from the same structure, the primordial phallus.** has one X chromosome, the second is replaced by a small stump, known as the Y chromosome – the male chromosome.

I don't want to alarm anyone, but the Y chromosome is the smallest of the chromosomes and it appears to be disappearing somewhat. Male fertility is therefore also in decline. That doesn't necessarily mean that men are going to die out, but nothing is impossible in the process of natural evolution.

So long as the Y chromosome does its work, we will continue to have men and their penises. It is precisely this small Y chromosome that sets a few major transformations into motion, by which an embryo can develop into a male.

The genetic blueprint for the genitalia can differ considerably from man to man, but your penis is probably around the average length of that of your closest relatives. Some families have longer penises on average, others have a shorter average length.

At least, that average length is in principle reached if the blueprint is followed correctly. That can only happen if the right substances are released in the right order. But things can go wrong.

The formation of the female sex organs is largely an automatic process. It happens naturally and no extra effort is required in girls. The phallus remains small in female foetuses and, for the most part, in the same place, between the legs. The labioscrotal swellings continue to consist of two separate halves. They become the labia majora, between which you find the vaginal opening.

Making a penis and scrotum from the same structures requires a lot of energy. The fact that you have a blueprint for a penis in your DNA doesn't automatically mean that you'll be born with a penis. Substances are needed to actively stimulate the building work. If that doesn't happen, the blueprints aren't followed, and the sex structures develop in the female way.

The substances that organise the building site of the male genitalia are the sex hormones. They are produced by the sex glands or gonads. In boys, the gonads develop into testicles under the influence of the Y chromosome; in girls, they become the ovaries. The testicles are therefore the building developer of the penis.

In boys, the phallus grows and becomes more prominent, and it holds the urethra within its structure. The labioscrotal swellings fuse together to become a pouch to hold the testicles in, once they are ready to descend from the abdominal cavity. The sex hormones testosterone and its derivative dihydrotestosterone are the drivers behind these transformations.

In addition to major building works, a male foetus also has a whole demolition process ahead. The anti-Müllerian hormone (AMH) is responsible for this. Under the influence of this 'anti-female hormone', the male foetus does away with the primordial female structures that every embryo has and which would otherwise grow into internal female sex organs, such as the vagina, womb and fallopian tubes.

A female foetus doesn't have the energy to waste on drastic renovation works. The primordial female sex organs continue to grow as usual and, in the absence of male hormones, the male structures dissolve spontaneously.

The entire development process of external and internal genitalia is especially complex and things can go wrong at every stage. The blueprint in the DNA needs to be right, the sex glands need to develop and produce hormones, parts that don't fit need to be got rid of. If things go wrong, this is when we see variations in sex development. This is the field of 'intersex' or 'differences in sex development' – one of my specialist areas as a urologist.

For example, there could be just one error in the DNA's genetic blueprint. Or, the DNA could be perfectly fine, with the correct blueprint for the penis and scrotum, but there is a problem with the hormones. Then the finishing work won't be right. Hormonal problems can be internal, i.e. caused by the foetus itself. But hormones from the mother or the environment can also throw a spanner in the works. Without **In extreme cases, a genetic girl can be born with a fully developed penis.** male hormones, the embryonic phallus automatically develops into a clitoris, and labia majora and minora grow, regardless of the DNA blueprint.

Some abnormalities are mild, others are very pronounced. The primordial gonads usually develop into ovaries or testicles, but sometimes you get a combination of both. Some patients have one ovary, half a vagina and half a womb on one side and one testicle with the vas deferens (tube that carries the sperm away) on the other.

We used to call these people 'true hermaphrodites'. That was a dreadful term, but it has been replaced by an equally dreadful one, namely 'a chromosomal ovotesticular disorder of sex development'.

In extreme cases, a genetic girl can be born with a fully developed penis, or a genetic boy can be born with a completely normal-looking female sex organ.

A condition exists where the body doesn't produce any dihydrotestosterone, the potent hormone that ensures men get a penis with a scrotum below. Without this hormone, you look like a female from the outside at birth, but inside you are male: you have testicles rather than ovaries. These testicles produce so much testosterone during puberty that you grow a beard and your voice breaks. Your testicles can descend into what look like labia majora from the outside. However, your penis doesn't develop any further – your external genitalia continue to look female.

This happened recently to two brothers from Iraq. Before puberty, they grew up as girls, but during puberty their bodies suddenly became very male. However, their genitalia didn't grow with them and continued to look female. Because of this, and also the dangerous situation in their country, the brothers fled and gained asylum in Belgium. Heads turn when they walk down the street, because they are very handsome men. They are currently receiving treatment from us. In a first stage we removed their female structures and created a micropenis from the clitoris. One year on we are doing a penis reconstruction or phalloplasty.

Your body can also be insensitive to the sex hormones, known as *androgen insensitivity syndrome* (AIS). This is where a person possesses external female genitals, because there is no action of testosterone to form a penis and a scrotum, but internal male gonads with no internal female structures. Belgian model Hanne Gaby Odiele is an example of someone with complete androgen insensitivity. Insensitivity can also be partial, for example people with a reasonably developed phallus and labia that have grown together. In such cases, the opening of the urethra is often on the underside of the penis.

The largest group of children with differences in sex development are girls whose adrenal glands don't produce enough cortisol because of an inherited disorder. Instead, their adrenal glands release a hormone with a similar effect to testosterone. The effects of this disorder are visible externally. Stimulated by the male hormones, the phallus grows into a reasonably large clitoris in mild cases, but it can also grow into a fully fledged penis. This penis can hold the urethra within it either completely or partially and can have a scrotum below, albeit without any testicles inside.

Genetically, they are very much girls: they have two X chromosomes and two ovaries. The other internal female structures are also present. Even though these girls have a penis, they also have a womb and vagina. The only difference is that their vagina doesn't open up to the 'outside world' but somewhere in the urethra. Later in life these patients will need surgery to bring the vagina down to the outer world in the perineum.

This inherited disorder can also occur in boys, although it doesn't affect their sex development.

Gender and social rigidity

Sex is dichotomous: you have a penis or a vagina. You are male or female. Only in a very small number of conditions does the external sex appear to be in two minds about which one they are. But just because someone has a penis it does not mean that they are by definition a *he*. If all you look at is the external sex organs, you don't know what's inside and much less how someone feels: male, female or something in between.

Around 15 years ago, a young woman was referred to me from Greece. She was about 18 years old and she came to me for a vaginal reconstruction. What she didn't know was that she was born a boy without a penis, a very rare disorder. The doctors immediately decided to remove her testicles to be sure that no male hormones could become active. They thought making 'him' a 'her' was the best option, and would allow her parents to bring her up as a girl. Later on, the girl needed a vagina made and she was sent to me for that very reason.

She herself was in no hurry for one. 'Do I really need a vagina?', she asked. 'Because I'm a lesbian.'

I was sitting opposite a heterosexual male who *thought* he was a lesbian. I sent her back to Greece with an urgent request to her doctors to explain everything to her fully. Unfortunately, I never saw the girl again and don't know what became of her.

The fact that differences in sex development can occur on so many levels explains why gender variance really isn't that rare. It affects one in every five thousand people, which is a considerable number of individuals. And that's not to mention transgenders.

Gender – our sexual identity, so to speak – is a lot more fluid than biological sex, with a whole spectrum of possibilities. Some very feminine homosexuals want to keep their penis and wouldn't dream of swapping it for a vagina. Whereas sex is very strongly influenced by hormones, gender is largely determined by our brain. But we still don't know where in our brain. There are differences in the layout of the brain, but also hormonal differences. Even aspects of upbringing can influence gender.

There are many people who don't identify themselves as 100 per cent male or female.

There are many people who don't identify themselves as 100 per cent male or female, without it being a problem. One and a half per cent of people feel very strongly that their sexual identity doesn't correspond with their biological sex. When their discomfort convinces them to seek treatment, they are given the diagnosis of gender dysphoria.

The extremely dichotomous view of the sexes stubbornly persists – 'You are the one and thus, by definition, not the other' – but this view is no longer sustainable. If you think back to the whole process of how the genitalia develop, it is clear that a whole range of variations are possible in the typical distinction of male/female. Variations can equally occur during the development of gender identity in our brain. We cannot cling on to that rigid distinction.

Because it is impossible to predict how a child will develop, it is best we don't try to put a child with a difference in sex development into a strict male or female category too early. I did that to patients myself 20 years ago and I've stopped doing it now.

It is true that you often feel a lot of pressure from the parents of a patient to do something. Such was the case with one pregnant mother whose non-invasive prenatal test (NIPT) showed she was having a girl. However, the ultrasound scan showed a penis. We knew before the birth that something wasn't right and, indeed, due to a hormonal problem the baby girl was born with a penis. Her parents were very keen for us to operate, because she had a womb and ovaries as well as a penis and scrotum. Why didn't we make her a girl straight away?

I stood by the bed of that child and thought: *Imagine if on her 18th birthday this girl feels transsexual and wants to be a boy. Then we will have to make her a penis, whereas hers was previously removed. We can never make a penis as good as the one she already has.*

The decisions we have to make are not easy. What are the rights of the parents and what are the rights of the child? I try to perform surgery in as few cases as possible without the child having the final say. But what if the parents really want a choice to be made? You can explain to them how a penis develops and why their child does or does not have one, but it is particularly hard to get people away from the idea that a boy should have a penis and a girl should not.

My belief is that the interest of the child is more important than social expectations. As a doctor, I always ask myself: *Will the patient actually be better off if I operate?*

A normal penis

Sex development can vary. But even when the penis has developed completely normally, they can vary in length and

15

width and all too quickly receive the stamp 'abnormal'. Most people aren't taught about the statistics and they hurry to see the doctor about penis 'abnormalities' that are statistically perfectly normal.

They might be worried about the length, the volume of sperm, or the number of times they have sex per week or month. When men see a urologist, they usually complain of their penis being 'too short' or 'too little'. They rarely complain that they ejaculate too much sperm or that their penis is too long. Only when they feel inadequate in one way or another do they say, 'Doctor, it's not normal.'

But what does 'normal' actually mean? Physical characteristics, such as penis length or volume of ejaculate, have a normal distribution and so 'normal' is not the opposite of 'abnormal'. 'Normal' is just a statistical term that describes the distribution of measurements. 'Normal distribution' looks like a bell curve, also known as the Gaussian curve, named after the nineteenth-century German mathematician Carl Gauss.

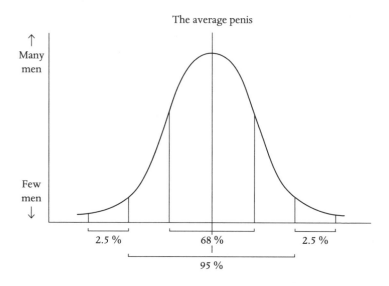

The figure makes one thing clear: the values coming in around the average are the most common. Most men, therefore, have an average-length penis, or ejaculate a quantity of sperm that's not far off the average. The more a value differs from the average, the less often it occurs. In other words: the longer or shorter a penis, the more uncommon it is.

The curve is symmetric: half of men have a penis that is smaller than average, the other half have a penis that is longer than average.

In order to find out the average penis length, we would have to measure the penis of every man in the world. That's just not possible. Therefore, we take random samples. The more men we select, the greater the chance of the measurements reflecting the general population.

The standard deviation is the figure which tells us how far you are from the average. If your penis length falls within one standard deviation, it is more or less the same length as the average. Sixty-eight per cent of men are in that category. Ninety-five per cent of all penises are a maximum of within two standard deviations of the average. This means that 2.5 per cent of men have a penis that is much shorter than the average, whereas, on the opposite end of the Gaussian curve, 2.5 per cent of penises are much longer than the average. Those are unusual measurements, but, statistically speaking, they still aren't abnormal.

So just how long is the average penis?

2

Penis length

Man and his oversized penis

The primary function of the penis is to serve as a reproductive organ. The fact that mammals also use their penis for the secondary function of urinating is simply a question of biological economy. Imagine you had two separate organs for disseminating your sperm and urinating: the two would just get in the way of each other. It is precisely to make internal fertilisation possible that the penis has a certain length.

Funnily enough, the average penis in humans is far longer than strictly necessary. Gorillas and chimpanzees do it with a lot less and they still manage to fertilise their females. When erect, a grown gorilla has a penis length of four centimetres, and a chimpanzee erection measures eight centimetres. With an average length of over 13 centimetres, humans outshine their close relatives.

What do we have to thank for the over-proportional size? Usually, natural selection does away with characteristics that don't serve a function – for example, the body hair that humans for the most part have lost. Things that aren't needed are done away with, because making excess tissue wastes energy.

So why does man have such a long penis?

The answer is because, alongside natural selection, there is another mechanism at play: sexual selection. Natural selection ensures that a species adapts optimally to its environment, sexual selection supplies the characteristics to give a species the greatest chance of mating. Therefore, sexual selection exaggerates some characteristics without natural selection undoing them. Think of the long, colourful tails of birds of paradise or peacocks. For one reason or another, female birds like a long tail, so a male with a long tail has more chance of reproducing, even if such an impractical attachment increases the risk of him being caught by a predator.

In the animal kingdom, we see an endless range of tactics for attracting potential partners. The huge chest muscles of male gorillas are another example. The male gorilla has an imposing presence, even though he only has a small penis. *Homo sapiens* generally flaunt a smaller muscular structure, but they have the largest penis of all primates, in terms of both proportion to body height and absolute length. This points to sexual selection.

Exactly how this came about in evolution, we don't know. There were no scientists around at the time observing primitive humans. We suspect the civilisation process played a role in it.

For a long time, man was a predator; a hunter-gatherer searching for food in the wild. Physical fitness was necessary to survive. At a certain time – or, even, over a period of time – humans became farmers. We took nature into our own hands and brute strength slowly lost importance. With farming, it wasn't about who could run fastest or jump furthest; it was who could produce the most from his land. The physical characteristics needed to impress females became less prominent. Perhaps that is why, as compensation, the penis grew bigger.

Coitus was a brief affair in primitive humans. There was no foreplay: humans lived in a threatening environment and men were well aware that others could be close by on the look-out for a woman who was ready for sex. The faster they could deposit their sperm, the better. And how did women know that a man was ready for sex? Attraction is a game of smell, pheromones, blushing cheeks and deep breathing, but the most important sign of arousal is the erection. Because sex had to take place so quickly, a large penis facilitated a quick selection.

Over time, humans started wearing clothes and that created a nice paradox: the very fact that humans were covering up their body made the penis more prominent. For that we have a muscle to thank that has since lost its function.

Most mammals have a layer of muscle under the skin. Horses, for example, can use it to twitch their skin to get rid of flies. Primitive humans could do that too. Now we only have the remains of such a muscle in the human body, for example in the groin, where we have the fascia of Scarpa. We also still have one of these superficial muscles in the neck, a small muscle in the hand, and a muscle in the skin of the scrotum and penis: the dartos muscle.

Most people with a penis have no idea that there is a muscle around their sex organ, because you can only see it if you look at the penis skin under a microscope. Men don't walk around displaying biceps in their penis, and the dartos muscle doesn't let you twitch your penis, either. So what does it do?

Not a single male mammal walks around waving its penis, apart from when a male feels a great desire to mate. In most mammals, the dartos muscle neatly tucks the flaccid penis inside the body. When *Homo sapiens* walked around naked, their penis was also hidden from view. When you're climbing over sharp rocks or running through thorny bushes, you want to keep your genitalia as close as possible to the body. Only with sexual arousal did the dartos muscle relax and the penis come out.

The muscle also runs as far as the skin of the scrotum, where it helps with the temperature regulation of the testicles. Each testicle is connected to a vas deferens which is also surrounded by a muscle. When the testicles get too warm, the vasa deferentia let the testicles hang down; if it suddenly gets cold, they tuck the testicles in. At the same time, the dartos muscle contracts the skin of the scrotum. That's why your penis looks small if you swim in cold water.

As people started to wear clothes, the purpose of this muscle diminished. Clothing took on its protective role, and men with a strong dartos muscle no longer had an evolutionary advantage from this. Natural selection did its work, but a redundant body part doesn't disappear in 20 or even 100 generations. In 10,000 years there have been around 330 generations, but the dartos muscle is still there.

It'll keep the penis company for a while longer, but it just does less than before. The penis and scrotum are no longer drastically drawn inside the body of modern man; at most they shrivel up a little.

Some men might be sorry that the dartos muscle is an involuntary muscle, over which they have no control. I can imagine that some would jump at the chance to make their penis look longer in a communal changing room. But, alas, the dartos muscle only relaxes at higher temperatures or in the case of moderate arousal. In the case of strong sexual arousal, the dartos muscle contracts again, to prepare for ejaculation. An erect penis doesn't decrease in size because of this, but the testicles are pressed closer to the body.

Two penises can be exactly the same length when erect, but the man with an active dartos muscle will appear to have the smallest penis when flaccid. He might think to himself about the other man: *Blimey, he's well hung!* But what he could perhaps think is: *Poor thing, he's got a bit of a lazy dartos muscle there!*

Therein lies the second paradox that burdens the male member. As I mentioned earlier, compared to other animals, men have an oversized penis. Because it also hangs outside the body, it catches the eye even more. So what do men do? They compare. And then all too quickly they come to the conclusion: *Oh no, mine is too small.*

Funnily enough, many men – and women – don't even know how long the average penis is.

The statistical penis

Take 1,000 men, undress them and give them an erection – you can use whichever method you want, it doesn't make any difference. Then measure all these erections and select 100 penises that measure exactly 13 centimetres. Stand these 100 men in a row and let their erection subside. Straight away, you will see vast differences in their penis lengths.

What can we conclude from this? That measuring penises isn't easy.

The only real measure for penis length is the length when extended. We take hold of the penis and extend it firmly. We then measure from the base (where it attaches to the abdomen) to the tip. The extended length (in medical literature this is named 'Stretched Penile Length', SPL) is the only objective basis for comparing penises. Now, the extended length barely differs from the erect length, but the temporary nature of an erection makes it impractical for large-scale scientific research. An erection also requires circumstances that conflict somewhat with the clinical world of science. Not many people get turned on by white coats and cold measuring instruments.

Warning! A whole load of figures now follow. But when I see how obsessed men are with the length of their penis, that might not be a bad thing.

The largest study on penis length dates from 2014. Data was collected from 15,521 men from all over the world, although the majority were white, with a minority of men of

African or Asian origin. This study showed that the average SPL is 13.2 centimetres. The average erect penis length is 13.12 centimetres. The average flaccid penis length is 9.16 centimetres.

Anything up to 1.5 centimetres above or below these figures is normal. In other words: 68 per cent of men have a flaccid penis length of between 7.59 and 10.73 centimetres; 95 per cent of men have a flaccid penis length somewhere between 6.02 and 12.3 centimetres. When erect, 68 per cent of men have a penis length of between 11.46 and 14.78 centimetres; 95 per cent of men have an erect penis length of between 9.8 and 16.44 centimetres.

So, now let's look at the exceptions. Only 2.5 per cent of men have a flaccid penis length of less than 6.02 centimetres and only 2.5 per cent of men have a flaccid penis length of more than 12.3 centimetres. Only 2.5 per cent of the population have an erection measuring less than 9.8 centimetres, and only 2.5 per cent of men have an erection measuring longer than 16.4 centimetres. Men falling into these categories have unusual lengths, but their penis is not abnormal.

The study also highlighted a few correlations between penis length and other physical characteristics. The most obvious one is the relation between length and width. A flaccid penis has an average circumference of 9.3 centimetres, the average circumference when erect is 11.6 centimetres – indeed, a lot more than you may have expected. Length and width usually correlate, so that a penis stays in proportion. Long narrow penises and short thick penises stand out: they are the exceptions.

There is also a correlation with ethnic origin. On the *World Map of Penis Size*, the average penis length differs depending on continent. In Africa, men originating from south of the Sahara usually have a longer penis than the world average. Men from East Asia have, on average, a shorter penis.

There are numerous theories on why these differences exist, but most of them aren't proven. Theories include, for example, the higher temperatures in Africa and the diet in East Asia, namely soya beans that contain a lot of oestrogen. However, these factors are far too weak. The most likely explanation is the difference in the genetic programme, the blueprint that determines what your penis looks like.

There is also a weak correlation between penis length and height: the taller the man, the greater the chance of him having a long penis. The same goes for BMI (*body mass index*, the relation between height and weight), where there is also a weak correlation. On this basis, the fatter the man, the greater the chance of him having a short penis. This is to do with the increased fat tissue at the base of the penis.

... if someone's ring finger is considerably longer than his index finger, there is a big chance he has a large penis.

There is no relation with the size of the feet, nose or ears. Penis length also bears no relation to finger length, although we do see a weak correlation between the ratio of the index finger to the ring finger. This phenomenon is known as the *digit ratio*. The index finger is usually shorter than the ring finger in both males and females, but the difference in length is greater in males. Exposure to male hormones before birth is said to determine that difference, just like hormones determine how big your penis becomes. One study showed that if someone's ring finger is considerably longer than his index finger, there is a big chance he has a large penis.

There is also an extremely weak link between penis length and anogenital distance – the distance between the back of the scrotum and the anus. In women, the anogenital distance is the distance between the anus and the vulva. Men usually have a larger anogenital distance. The same applies here too: more male hormones increase the anogenital distance, as well as penis length. However, testicle volume doesn't appear to bear any relation to penis length.

Another weak link is age. As men age, they lose muscle strength and elasticity, including of the dartos muscle, which draws the genitalia closer towards the body. The longer gravity does its work, the less resistance the dartos muscle provides, and the lower the penis and scrotum hang.

In some birth defects, we see an enormous difference in the organisation of the dartos muscle, but the muscle also makes the penis length constantly vary in normal individuals too. Sometimes it contracts less, sometimes more. When men compare their penises in a flaccid state, the difference can largely be attributed to the activity of the dartos muscle at that particular time. This is another reason why the SPL is the correct way to measure the penis. Anything in the range of 13 centimetres is completely normal.

If, for whatever reason, you are on the look-out for an above-average penis size, then you should look in the direction of a tall slim black man with a very long ring finger and a large distance between the back of his scrotum and his anus. Based on the statistics, this type of person is your best bet, but remember that statistical probability doesn't always correlate with reality.

So, we now know what the average penis length is, but does scientific research also tell us what the *ideal* penis is? Yes it does. The answer is simple: any penis that is long and hard enough to penetrate the vagina and deliver sperm inside. To that end, most men walk around with an ideal penis. Provided it is sensitive enough and your partner gets pleasure from it, the world is a perfect place.

If your number-one desire is to give women sexual pleasure, then penis length itself comes second to penis width. Women's genital sensitivity is mainly – although not exclusively – located at the entrance to the vagina, so a wide penis stimulates the labia minora and clitoris more than a narrow one does. Therefore, it doesn't matter if the penis is shorter or longer than average. Only if a penis is too short to reach the entrance to the vagina is length a problem.

Unfortunately, many men don't see it that way. They compare their penis with other penises in a flaccid, non-extended state and then draw all kinds of conclusions that have no statistical or biological basis. You can tell them a hundred times that their penis is completely within the normal range, but in their eyes it will always be too small.

In today's porn culture, the importance of a long penis is still over-emphasised, but the penises you see in porn films are two standard deviations from the norm. That is statistical jargon to say the penises you see in porn films are unusually big. The lengths seen in barely 2.5 per cent of men simply can't be considered the norm.

The small end of the spectrum

If men wonder why their penis looks a certain way, the answer usually lies in the DNA they inherited from their parents. If you have a relatively small penis, there is a high chance that your dad has a similar looking weapon in his trousers. The fact of the matter is: penis length is programmed in the DNA.

The programme in the genes determines the design and the hormones ensure the blueprint is followed. All this happens before you are even born. Every embryo starts off with all male and female characteristics to begin, but boys' hormones need to work hard to develop the male structures effectively and get rid of the female ones. Development happens as good as automatically in girls, but male hormones need to continually tell the boy's body to grow the primordial phallus into a penis and fuse together the labia to produce a pouch to hold the testicles.

Mini-puberty begins about three months after birth. At that point, hormones from the testicles give the penis a new growth spurt. After mini-puberty, the penis usually grows in line with the body, so that everything stays more or less in proportion. The average extended penis length of a young child is about four centimetres. It won't get much longer until puberty.

When puberty comes, the penis suddenly seems to grow exponentially. A new surge of male hormones can make it grow up to three times bigger – a growth that our body isn't used to. That's the *big shot*, the big leap forwards.

Or, at least, that's the aim. Sometimes the DNA has a programme for a normal penis, but something goes wrong hormonally and no, or too few, hormones are produced. Or all the building components are there, but the body doesn't respond to them – a typical example of this is androgen insensitivity syndrome.

Think of hormones as keys that fit into a keyhole, the receptor. Normally, there are an equal number of keys and keyholes. However, sometimes you can have enough keys, but not enough keyholes. In this case, your hormones don't kick in, and your penis turns out smaller than the blueprint intended. If you don't have any keyholes at all, a penis simply won't grow.

Some infants have a penis measuring less than 1.5 centimetres. We call this a micropenis. We can give these boys additional hormonal stimulation to make their penis grow longer. Then their penis reaches the length it would have been at puberty a few years earlier. You can argue that there is no point in this; however it is a kind of psychological protection. It ensures that these boys don't have anything to be ashamed of in the changing room. During puberty, their penis will grow less than their peers, but that's 12 years down the line.

We don't have enough good measurements of penis length to look back over hundreds of years, but some think that penises appear to be getting shorter worldwide. Perhaps environmental factors play a role in this, because we are seeing a slight decrease in penis length in the industrialised world in particular.

A possible cause are the hormone disruptors that are increasingly appearing in the environment. They not only reduce fertility but impede penis growth too. The decrease isn't dramatic, but it exists. The fact that the reduced penis length has been observed mainly in alligators in Florida shouldn't stop us from taking it seriously: if alligators are susceptible to hormone disruptors, there's no reason to think that humans are immune.

... some think that penises appear to be getting shorter worldwide. Perhaps environmental factors play a role in this.

Hormone disruptors get into the environment through pesticides, for example. Or just think about all that plastic that makes its way into the natural world. And then there's the contraceptive pill. It has been around since 1950, and since then not a single pill has remained in a woman's body. The pill is made from artificially manufactured female hormones and the body doesn't break them down completely. They get into the environment via urine and waste water. It is very difficult to eliminate these hormones and, unfortunately, it is even more difficult to establish to what extent these hormones are being spread around.

We are starting to see a similar effect in hormonally stimulated pregnancies. There appear to be more birth defects affecting the penis in such pregnancies than in natural, spontaneous pregnancies. You may be stimulating fertility, but sabotaging the penis.

Fortunately, there is a placenta separating the unborn child from the outside world. This keeps many substances at bay that could potentially shorten the penis. Our own research at Ghent University Hospital has shown that placental abnormalities cause more penis defects in boys. And once you are born, the placenta no longer protects you, leaving you exposed to all kinds of influences.

Even if the penis's genetic blueprint is strictly followed and you should in principle have an impressive sex organ to flaunt, another deal-breaker can come along: the dartos muscle.

I explained earlier that this muscle shrinks the scrotum and draws the penis inside in most mammals. Modern man lost the function of this muscle to some extent when he began to wear clothes. If you're wearing trousers, there's less risk of your crown jewels getting caught on thorny bushes, after all.

However, man still has this muscle, and some people have a more active muscle than others. Cases of the *disappearing penis* have been reported in Japan, where the dartos muscle of patients with a certain form of psychosis tucks the penis completely inside. In another form of psychosis, men are overwhelmed by the fear that their penis will disappear and it is exactly this fear itself that makes the dartos muscle contract, actually making their penis 'disappear'.

Another condition is the *buried penis*, where the penis appears to be completely buried inside the body. That too, among other things, is down to a dartos muscle contracting excessively, but this time without a psychological factor playing a part. Of all the mothers who have come to me asking whether their baby's penis is too small, more than half were cases of a buried penis. (The other half were mothers who didn't know what normal was and were comparing their sons to babies who happened to be very well hung.)

Every year, we perform a good 20 operations to remove the dartos muscle from the penis, so that it can no longer draw the penis inside. We do not know the cause of this condition.

It is possible that hormone disruptors have something to do with this too.

You can also 'bury' your penis with an unhealthy lifestyle. Obesity is one of the major causes of penises looking smaller. Losing 10 kilograms or so instantly gives the penis an extra centimetre in length. If you want a good reason to lose some excess weight, that has to be one.

Finally, your penis can become shorter following surgery. Men who have their prostate removed end up with a smaller penis. The prostate, the gland that produces up to a third of seminal fluid, surrounds the urethra. When the prostate is removed, the urethra becomes five centimetres shorter and therefore the penis loses some of its length, too.

Also, when men come to us asking us to straighten their curved penis, we unfortunately have to tell them that they will end up with a shorter penis. In a curved penis, the two columns of erectile tissue are unequal in length, and so we shorten the longest of the two. This makes the penis straighter, but also shorter.

It is a question of deciding: straighter or longer? If your curved penis doesn't affect your sex life and isn't painful, it's sometimes better just to leave it as it is.

Having the biggest

No man feels offended if you suggest he has a small liver. Mumble under your breath something about a small penis and you awaken the gorilla in him. The penis of a presidential candidate even came up during the 2016 US elections.

One of Donald Trump's opponents, Republican Marco Rubio, drew attention to Trump's small hands. He added, 'You know what they say about men with small hands...'

Trump couldn't let that go. He tried every defence to refute the allegation – not once, but multiple times. Even he knew a superpower like the US couldn't be led by someone with a small penis. What good are all those missiles and atomic bombs if the president is lacking down below?

During one debate, Trump held up his hands. 'Look at those hands,' he said to the audience. 'Are they small hands? If they're small, something else must be small. I guarantee you there's no problem. I guarantee.'

Trump was elected as president and it was only after the elections that we learned more about his penis. Porn actress Stormy Daniels claimed she had sex with the then presidential candidate and, in her memoir, she disclosed the details the whole world was waiting to hear: the length of the president's manhood. According to her, it was small but 'not freakishly small'. She considered it 'smaller than average', but **Losing 10 kilograms or so instantly gives the penis an extra centimetre in length.** let's assume that the average penis a porn actress encounters is somewhat bigger than the scientifically established average. Unfortunately, mediocrity is also problematic for someone who describes all his merits in the superlative.

So why do we attach so much importance to penis size? It tells us nothing about someone's intelligence or qualities as a leader. So long as a penis does what it needs to do – deliver sperm into the vagina and pass urine out of the body – penis length is of no relevance. It's not penis length that will win over women – by the time a woman wants to see your penis, she will probably already have fallen for other characteristics of your body or personality.

People continue to associate a large penis with high fertility. In reality that association doesn't exist, but we continue to think it. Therefore, the importance of a large penis is always magnified, just as goddesses of fertility always have huge breasts. We can't get away from the phallus's heritage of human culture and that culture comes partly from our genes. Our DNA is full of world history and it doesn't lie awake at night thinking that man has since invented the wheel, the combustion engine and the smartphone.

Times change more quickly than our DNA evolves, and our DNA still holds gorilla tendencies. A gorilla makes a lot of noise and shows off his muscles, actions that are recognizable in some *Homo sapiens* specimens. Men usually build their muscles not to lift heavy objects but to show them off. There is another dimension too when it comes to these muscles and which doesn't concern the gorilla: the cliché continues to exist that a tall, muscular man is well hung between his legs.

Sometimes that holds true, but more often than not it doesn't. Men who frequently work out at the gym and take pills to look big and strong end up with small testicles.

It's not women who fixate on the male crotch, but men themselves. If men think they don't have enough in their pants, they worry that this will be noticed. The truth is if they are being looked at at all, it's not by women but by other men, because women look at the whole body, not just the crotch. Penis length plays a role in situations where men find themselves temporarily undressed, for example in sports changing rooms. This is where men establish the pecking order based on penis size.

Men with a long penis like to prance around with it hanging out. They won't hide it away in these places because a large penis puts you higher up the hierarchical ladder. So macho men like to show theirs off, unless they come from Turkey or Morocco, for example. Many Muslims still prefer to shower in their underpants, regardless of their penis size. In general, men who are on the slightly smaller side will also hide theirs away. Likewise if they have a completely normal penis, but think theirs is smaller than average.

And thus they create a self-fulfilling prophecy: if men think they are on the small side, they also behave like they are lower down the pecking order.

Men who really want a longer penis almost always believe an oversized penis is a godsend. However, having an excessively long penis is no picnic for women. A long, wide penis may give your bed partner some extra stimulation, but there are limits. The vagina doesn't go on for ever. If a long penis reaches the cervix, it can push the womb upwards into the abdominal cavity. That kind of stimulation is unpleasant, if not painful.

A very long penis has a higher chance of being bent. A curved penis is usually the result of a difference in size between the two main columns of erectile tissue (*corpora cavernosa*). With a long penis, even a minimum difference between these corpora has a far greater effect, making the curvature more obvious.

The risk of injury also increases with length. That's a question of physics. During sex, you probably have other things on your mind than the lever principle, but that's exactly what is at play here. With a long penis, the forces exerted on the load arm are greater, resulting in more likelihood of a penile fracture than with a short penis.

That is pure physics, albeit with terribly painful consequences. Humans don't have any bones in their penis that can break, but the tube of solid tissue around the erectile tissue (which we call *tunica albuginea*) can tear. Such a tear doesn't go unnoticed. You hear a crunching noise, feel a sharp pain and your erection disappears. It quickly swells up purplish-blue and starts to resemble an aubergine. The term 'penile fracture' at least sounds as painful as this trauma feels. I'll give you a tip: the missionary position is the safest – avoid positions that exert a lot of sideways pressure, like the Amazon position with the woman on top.

A long length also disturbs the erection's hydraulic mechanism. Men with an exceptionally long penis (the 2.5 per cent with the biggest examples) sometimes suffer from inadequate erections because the pump system fails. The penis won't stick up and won't get hard, making penetration difficult. If your penis is so long that it doesn't work properly, you're not benefiting much from those extra few centimetres.

It's true that I don't hear many complaints about penises being too long: men very rarely go to the doctor's complaining of this. I've only encountered it three times in my whole career. As we've seen, if men worry about anything, it's about *lacking* in length.

The issue of having a larger penis exists all over the world, but it appears to be more prominent in Europe and the United States – however, that impression might have been distorted because there are more scientific journals on those continents.

'Ladies, if you see a man in his birthday suit and you think, "What a small penis", well, by all means think it, but never say it. Never.'

I believe many men deep down are not happy with their penis length. Too many men go to see a doctor about their small penis. And that's just those who have mustered enough courage to go. A lot more men stay at home, troubled about their sex organ and making the problem even worse.

When a man comes to an appointment with his – supposedly – small penis, a traumatic experience is usually the cause of his concerns. Some mothers tell their sons, 'You mustn't take off your *underpants* in the changing room.' They mean well – they don't want their son to be laughed at – but they are creating a problem and triggering anxiety. This boy is getting the message very early on: *you have a small penis, hide it away.*

If an insecure man gets a comment about his penis at the gym or in the bedroom, that can pretty much sour his relationship with his sex organ for good. I'm therefore forever drilling into my students: 'Ladies, if you see a man in his birthday suit and you think, *"What a small penis"*, well, by all means think it, but never say it. Never.' The anxiety that ensues from this is often the biggest reason why a man worries about his penis. Only once does a woman have to say, 'My, what a small penis you've got', and that man will spend the rest of his life perturbed by one careless utterance.

Some men have a penis that measures 14 centimetres when erect. However, when flaccid, the cold or stress can activate the dartos muscle and reduce its size to somewhere in the region of five centimetres. If someone happens to comment on your penis at that particular point in time, that's really unfortunate. You don't reply, 'Its statistically longer than average when in full action!' Instead, you cringe and start to worry.

Close-fitting sweatpants reveal everything, but some men have a complex about not filling their trousers with their too small bulge. They think everyone is looking at them because their penis isn't big enough. However, the reality is quite different: because they're scared that others are looking at them, they then begin to imagine that everyone is always looking at them, when it's simply not the case.

This kind of trauma can take dramatic forms. Some men have a perfectly normal penis and still believe it is far too small. These men suffer from PDD (penile dysmorphic disorder). There is a disparity between what they see and what is actually there. The patient sees something abnormal between his legs; his doctor sees nothing but a completely normal penis. The actual condition isn't in their trousers but rather in the patient's head.

Men with PDD can no longer see their penis in the right proportions. It's not entirely illogical: if you look at your penis from above, you're looking from the wrong direction. It makes your penis look shorter than it actually is. In the changing rooms, men look at other penises from the correct angle – and mainly at the ones that stand out. And then they compare the false image they have of their penis with the exceptions that are bigger than the norm. When they try to measure their penis, they use the wrong method and the wrong benchmarks to compare. They receive an influx of false information that convinces men with a normal penis that theirs is too small.

Your crotch is irrelevant in normal, daily life. In the context of sexual arousal, a woman might take a look at what's hanging or standing between your legs, but outside the bedroom nobody is bothered about your crotch. However, for men who are worried about theirs, it is extremely relevant.

Treating PDD is difficult, very difficult even. Men who suffer from it just can't rid themselves of their delusion. It's almost like a mini-psychosis. I often hear the female partner say, 'How is it possible? Everything's great for me, but my partner is obsessed with his penis all day.'

A man who fixates on this is in big trouble, because there isn't a single solution for the lack of length that bothers him so. You can show him the world map of penis length (which you can google and find online) a hundred times, explain how the Gaussian curve works and stress to him that his penis length is statistically perfectly normal, but it won't make any difference.

Many of these men ask for an operation, but surgery isn't the right way to solve the problem. Those who undergo surgery often end up with a disfigured penis. No single procedure can make your penis longer without damaging it.

Why would you let your penis be maimed while women don't pay that much attention to it? Research shows it is not the crotch that women look at when they are searching for a partner.

Women look at other things

Ancient Greek athletes performed completely naked and, yes, they felt shy about their penis. A glans penis (the rounded head or tip of the penis) peeping out could be quite embarrassing for its bearer. To prevent this from happening, the athletes tied a leather strip known as a *kynodesme* around their foreskin. This kept the head of the penis safely inside. One can only imagine what it would have been like to be wrestling in the dust with another naked opponent, never mind with the head of your penis suddenly exposed for all to see.

There are men in our modern-day changing rooms who no longer have a foreskin left to tie. Their glans penis is open and exposed at the end of their penis. They only feel shame if they think their penis is too small, whereas the Ancient Greeks considered 'retractivity' to be an advantage.

Men who have been favourably endowed sometimes assume that their large penis is a VIP pass: not only does their penis rank them higher in the pecking order, they only have to show their erection to a woman for her to fall at their feet in wonder.

Well, the reality can be quite disappointing. How so? It comes down to the vagina.

The seventeenth century Dutch anatomist Reinier de Graaf was the first to praise the vagina. He said, 'The length of the penis isn't important, because the vagina adapts to anything.' The female pelvic floor muscles are indeed a powerful organ; they help increase the contact between the genitals.

Because the vagina adapts so easily to the penis penetrating it, differences in penis length really don't matter so much. A woman will feel extra stimulation from a very wide penis, but whether a penis is a few centimetres longer or shorter is of no importance.

Thanks to scientific research, we know that women don't judge a man by the size of his crotch. Female research subjects were given a pair of glasses to wear that monitored their eye movements and were then asked to look at men. The conclusion? Women look at men's shoulders and thighs, their butt and their muscles, and only then, last of all, do their eyes turn to the trouser bulge. While an awful lot of men think that everything pivots around their crotch, women are generally more interested in the overall appearance of a man.

Back when humans didn't wear clothes, the erect penis came in handy to seduce a potential partner, but since we have been wandering the earth wearing clothes, other symbols have replaced the role of the penis. In the present day, men rely on their Porsche or Ferrari, for example.

Because men continue to associate a big penis with sexual power, penis length plays a big role within gay culture, or, in any case, a far greater role than with heterosexuals. While it's true there are a lot of homosexuals who are less concerned about that side of things, in a certain niche of the gay environment, generally men quickly drop their gaze on to the crotch of potential sexual partners.

... gay men with a small penis are *penalised* twice, both socially and sexually.

With undue importance being placed on penis length, gay men with a small penis are *penalised* twice, both socially and sexually. They too suffer from the changing-room syndrome – they are ashamed of their penis and worry they will topple down the hierarchical ladder. Not to mention that finding a sexual partner will be more difficult. This isn't right for these poor men, but it's down to a deep-routed biological programme that makes you feel more relaxed and comfortable assuming you will be more successful and powerful with a big penis.

It's even more complex with trans men. When you change a female body into a male body, you have to decide whether to make a small but fully sensitive penis out of the clitoris, or whether to create a long but less sensitive penis using phalloplasty. For some, size matters most. In anticipation of the operation, these men walk around with a rubber penis down their trousers, getting themselves and their scene used to their filled crotch.

No, it won't get any longer

There are people who can acquire a reasonably long penis by surgical means, but these are mostly trans men. They are born in a female body, with female genitalia, but they feel male. To give these transsexual men a penis, we normally use phalloplasty. We take a flap of skin from the arm, roll it up and sew it to the part of the body where the penis belongs. This gives them a penis measuring about 13 centimetres long. It can be inflated using a penile implant.

Some boys are born without a penis (for example in the case of penile agenesis, which is a rare congenital disease affecting 1 in 250,000 male newborns), while others lose their penis in an accident. Phalloplasty is also the answer in those cases. But using phalloplasty in biological men with a completely normal penis? Sorry, but I don't agree with that. I don't believe in sacrificing a small 'real thing' for a big 'lookalike'.

Not long ago, a 17-year-old boy came for a consultation. He had driven to Ghent from Bordeaux in France. He found his penis too small because of a rare congenital disease called bladder exstrophy. This is where the bladder and urethra are open to the outer world and which presents with a short, open penis, which we close surgically. His doctors had referred him to me, saying, 'Go to Ghent, I'm sure they'll find a solution there.'

When extended, his penis was seven centimetres long and he was hoping for phalloplasty. In other words, to cut off his real penis and replace it with a rolled-up flap of skin from his arm. I had to disappoint the young man.

'There's no way I can replace your functional penis with one that doesn't work as well,' I told him.

He wouldn't accept that. I had to explain in every way I could that he didn't have a problem that merited an operation. 'You have a very wide penis,' I said. 'That is an *advantage*, even if the length is relatively short.'

Being laughed at in the sports club fills your mind with the idea that your penis is inadequate. It's a serious matter and I understand how this can torment men. But the fact that there are professionals out there who would advise a young man like that to have surgery is too crazy for words. These people are giving the message, 'Yes, your penis is too short, get it replaced.' They are just creating an even bigger problem.

A penis is not there to make an impression in the changing room, but to give pleasure in bed. A wide penis measuring seven centimetres in length does not stand in the way of that pleasure. That's what those doctors should have told the young man. There is absolutely no reason to sacrifice a functional, sensitive penis for a less sensitive look-alike that can't get a spontaneous erection.

A penis is not there to make an impression in the changing room, but to give pleasure in bed.

A too-small penis is, more than anything, an imaginary problem. It can of course adversely affect your social life by making you avoid certain situations, but rarely is there something medically wrong. Only if your penis is less than six centimetres long (a micropenis) do you really have a problem, because you can't penetrate a woman and it will be difficult to get her pregnant.

The worst thing of all is that we cannot help such men with a micropenis. Again and again, we have to repeat our most important message: you can't make your penis much longer without damaging it. Unfortunately, obscure websites promise the opposite, tempting you to pay for all kinds of appliances, pills and massage techniques. None of this rubbish actually makes your penis any longer.

Even the swimwear industry takes advantage of our obsession with having the biggest. You can now buy swimming trunks with extra filling, to make you look bigger. In the eighties we wore shoulder pads to give us broad shoulders – now we are doing the same with the penis.

Padded swimming trunks are really quite innocent, however, when you see what instruments of torture are offered to men on the internet! One example is the 'penis stretcher', a double clamp to stretch your penis. It is absurd that someone would want to walk around wearing that all day. The sales pitch claims that the permanent tension encourages your cells to divide, creating more tissue mass. Nonsense. What the device does is wear out the dartos muscle so your penis looks a bit longer at rest.

A penis stretcher can easily cost 200 euros and you are definitely being swindled. The reviews of dissatisfied customers don't lie: 'It is painful.' 'The thing doesn't stay on.' 'It is highly visible under clothes.' And above all: 'No results after four months!' The manufacturers claim that their stretcher increases the total length of the penis, but the truth is as soon as you stop wearing it, it will go back to its previous length.

Less painful is botulinum toxin, better known by the brand name Botox. Botox is mainly used to reduce the appearance of facial wrinkles, but you can also inject it into the skin of the penis to paralyse the dartos muscle. For three months, this then gives you the same effect as a penis stretcher. If I wanted a villa in Saint Tropez, all I'd have to do is hang a sign above my front door saying: 'Botox penis extensions'. I offered Botox once and stopped right away. A patient kept repeatedly coming for a consultation asking me to make his penis longer. Because I was so tired of it I gave in and injected Botox. The results were short-lasting. After three months the effect was gone, and I didn't feel like injecting a series of men with Botox into their penises four times a year. As a doctor, you have to ask yourself why you are treating the penis cosmetically without there being a medical need.

But there are surgeons out there who promise perfectly healthy patients a longer penis. You mustn't believe these people and please don't let them mess with yours. Not so long ago, I saw a patient who had been operated on by a plastic surgeon in a hospital in Brussels. He had cut through the ligament which holds the penis close to the pubic bone and injected fat into it to make the penis thicker. The result? The patient was in quite a panic.

When erect, his penis pointed downwards and the fat injection meant his sex organ looked out of proportion. We removed the fat and repaired the ligament. The man had paid 9,000 euros for that penis. And he still wasn't happy.

95 per cent of men regret opting for a surgical penis extension.

And he is no exception: 95 per cent of men regret opting for a surgical penis extension. Perhaps the 5 per cent who are happy paid so much for the procedure that they can't bear to admit they've been duped!

The only thing we can do is prescribe adolescents with penile dysmorphic disorder a low dose of an erection-promoting drug. This gives them a continuous mild erection, which stretches the penis slightly. This can help men get over their shame or anxiety. However, we can't prescribe a pill to every man who thinks his penis is too small. Your social life and emotional well-being must be significantly impaired by it.

The best solution is to consult a sex therapist and learn to accept your body the way it is. That's not easy, but it's the healthiest option in the long term. I always say to my patients who have to go through life with a small penis, 'If your partner leaves you because of your penis, then they weren't worthy of your love and trust, and they didn't like you anyway.'

I know that's a cliché, but it's extremely important that young men find trust in their relationship. A penis, no matter how big or small, is only a tiny part of a good relationship. 'Learn to live with it,' is my message.

Some men with a small penis bring their girlfriend along to the consultation. The girlfriends are often very positive about their relationship and sex life. These men's problems exist more in their head than in their trousers.

It's all in the proportions

One of the most famous penises in the world can be visited in Florence. The penis belongs to a Jewish man, but his foreskin is still intact. What strikes admirers of Michelangelo's *David* more than anything is that he only has a small one. 'He felt threatened and this made his penis small,' some reason. Indeed, David was about to go to war with the giant Goliath.

Is David's penis really so small? The genius of Michelangelo is that the small penis doesn't stand out when you look at the statue from the right angle. The fact that David's thumb is twice as long as his penis is no mistake in the proportions. Quite the opposite: if David's hands were smaller and his penis were larger, we would be perturbed by the disproportion.

Proportions aren't just important in art: our brain also knows instantly if someone's body doesn't look right. Therefore, the most important characteristic of a penis is not so much that it is long, but that it is in proportion. A long narrow penis stands out just as much as a short wide penis: such proportions deviate from what we are used to.

People often underestimate penis width. The average circumference of a flaccid penis is nine centimetres; when erect it can go up to 11 centimetres, almost the same as the length.

Does this width have a function? No. At least, not for conceiving. However, as we've already seen, width does play a role in the sexual satisfaction of a female partner. A woman has more genital sensitivity at the outer edge of the vagina than deep within, as a lot of men incorrectly believe. A wide penis stimulates the sensitive areas better, making it easier for a woman to orgasm than with a long thin penis.

You can do as little about penis width as you can about penis length. Procedures *are* possible, but the results are shocking. Some patients have their penis injected with fat or, worse still, with Vaseline. That's very popular in Bulgaria. I would strongly advise anyone against even thinking about such a procedure. Vaseline in your penis is an abomination. Your body reacts badly to it and it is a terrible material to get rid of. Your penis no longer looks like a normal penis either, all proportionality is gone.

From a purely visual perspective, the ideal penis is one that *doesn't* stand out on a naked man, precisely because it is in proportion.

To ensure that the width of a penis is in optimal proportion to its length, the penis itself must be in proportion with the rest of the body. A very small penis doesn't fit with a very tall man, just as a very long penis looks wrong on a short man. If it doesn't fit, it looks wrong.

Some men having phalloplasty choose to use a flap of skin from their leg instead of their arm. That's what we do if they want a large, wide penis. However, we tell them that their penis might be out of proportion with the rest of their body.

An American urologist once operated on a young boy whose father had driven over him with a lawnmower. Exactly how that happened, you don't want to know, but the result was that this boy lost his penis. He was just a young child.

The doctor took a flap of skin from the boy's upper arm, made a penis out of it and sewed it on. 'Good job,' you might think. But the result sucked. The young boy had a penis that hung down to his knees.

It is precisely because proportionality is so important that we don't perform phalloplasty in children. The flap doesn't grow with the rest of you, so you start off with a penis that is far too big and end up with one that is too small.

From a purely visual perspective, the ideal penis is one that *doesn't* stand out on a naked man, precisely because it is in proportion.

Creative and diverse

I work with men who have a micropenis. A penis measuring five centimetres when erect is really very small. I nevertheless advise these men against phalloplasty because the results look like a penis and work like a penis, but they aren't a penis. I say to these patients, 'This is what you have to understand. Even with a small penis, you can experience a lot of pleasure.'

I don't know about everyone, but of the men who come to see me with a small penis, there are quite a few who sit in the corner scared and consumed with doubt.

How do you overcome that? Not so much with surgery, I believe, but with reassuring conversations. The ultimate way to overcome the problem is with a good relationship. Nevertheless, men in such a relationship still carry on hoping for a bigger penis, as though one fine day they will wake up with one. The ideal image of a big penis is deep-rooted in our minds.

You won't see a small penis appear in your average sex film. And so pornography upholds man's primitive feeling that length matters. Small men feel excluded and men with large penises stand out most, so you worry even more about your length. Men who feel their penis is too small don't need surgery, however, but advice from a sex therapist.

A bit of creativity in the bedroom can totally compensate for a so-called shortcoming in length. I'm not a sex therapist, but that's the message I often give men who worry about their penis size.

A small penis doesn't stand in the way of sexual pleasure. I know men with a micropenis who have particularly good sex lives. Getting this turnaround in a patient is difficult, but extremely important.

Some trans men don't want phalloplasty and opt for metoidioplasty instead, where we make a micropenis out of a clitoris. Trans men who opt for a micropenis retain both their natural erection – so they don't need an erectile prosthesis with a pump – and their sensation, after surgery. You can't penetrate your partner with a micropenis, but all the other pleasurable things are still possible. These men can live very happily with the fact that their penis is smaller than average: the quality of their sex lives is the benchmark, not the length of their penis. Many of these patients are quite satisfied – and if they aren't, phalloplasty is always an option.

Naturists have got over the belief that a long penis is the only 'right' kind of penis.

The reality of sex is that we really don't do it as often as we think and our daily sex lives really aren't as varied as the Kama Sutra. Most people on average make do with the same position: the missionary position. We often aren't very creative, but everyone – whether your penis is long or short – has the potential to enjoy a more creative sex life.

Introducing more creativity into the bedroom is one strategy for accepting your penis length. Another is to stop comparing your penis with false reference material. Pornography conveys a distorted image of what the average penis looks like. If all you see is huge penises, you're automatically going to believe that yours is exceptionally small. If you take a look at the real world, you will quickly realise that yours isn't so abnormal after all.

So where can you find the diversity of the real world? On a nudist beach or in a naked sauna. There you can see all the various forms that bodies can take. This gives you a far more realistic basis with which to compare your own body.

Naturists have got over the belief that a long penis is the only 'right' kind of penis. These people have overcome the uncertainty surrounding their body. Precisely by being so exposed among each other, they have a clearer picture of what normal is. By normalising nakedness again, you can accept your differences more easily. On the Dutch nudist beaches, where women sit knitting scarves, penis length is of no importance. Being naked among other people, without the context of seduction or sexuality, is a very healthy thing to do.

For men who are worried about their penis length, this is perhaps the healthiest tip of all: take yourself to places where there are penises of all sizes and where it simply doesn't matter who has the biggest.

Healthy mind, healthy penis

A healthy body means a healthy penis. Health won't make it longer, but a healthy penis will at least preserve its length. You also need to be mentally fit and healthy for your penis to be fit and healthy. If you're not, your penis isn't healthy and it will decrease in size.

Penile dysmorphic disorder can make you depressed and you end up in a vicious circle. Men who take antidepressants over a long period of time complain of their penis getting shorter, and they are right. Antidepressants decrease the number of erections a man has. This shrinks your penis, because spontaneous night-time erections are gymnastics for the penis. When your penis swells up often enough, it retains its length better.

Men battling with impotence have the same problem: they get fewer night-time erections, their penis gets less exercise and it becomes shorter.

So how do you know exactly how long your penis is? First of all, you need to measure it correctly and this can be done in various ways. Doing it yourself isn't difficult; you don't need to be a trained urologist. You can use an old-fashioned ruler or, if you prefer, a measuring app on your smartphone. The most important thing is that you know what you are supposed to be measuring. You start with the top, the side of the penis that you see. We want to measure the length from the point where the penis leaves the body to its tip.

If you're using a ruler, make sure it starts at 0 at the end – some rulers have a one centimetre margin. Watch out for that, otherwise your penis will instantly be one centimetre shorter! Then carefully measure the central axis of the penis.

If you decide to use the *augmented reality* ruler on your smartphone, you need to hold your penis nice and horizontally to measure it correctly – your penis should be at a 90-degree angle from your body. Make sure that the starting point of the measurement is the point where your penis leaves your body. If you have a lot of foreskin that goes beyond the tip of the glans (penis head), you can include this in your measurement.

If you want to know the length of your flaccid penis, think about the ambient conditions. The temperature should be optimal – if it's cold, the effect can be like a cold shower. Ideally, find somewhere that's nice and warm. It's best not to choose a time when you're very stressed either.

The exercise is a lot simpler with an erect penis. Your penis length stays constant for as long as the erection lasts. If you're using your smartphone, once again make sure your penis is at a 90-degree angle from your body – your smartphone doesn't have a perspective of depth.

If you're too stressed to measure your penis when erect, the maximum extended length is a suitable alternative. This is the method that urologists use during consultations. Hold your penis by its head and extend it as far as it will go. The principle is the same: you measure from the base to the tip. The extended length gives you an idea of the erect length, and an erection gives you a few millimetres more. If your extended length is 13.5 centimetres, your erect length is highly likely to be more than 14 centimetres.

Whatever the result, don't let it get to you. And although it isn't an exact science, I say it again: the happier you are, the fitter your penis. If you're depressed, your penis will be depressed and it will hide away in a corner.

3

The foreskin

A sensitive postcard

Once upon a time, thousands of years ago, humans started removing the foreskin. You may wonder why on earth they did that. The foreskin is not just an excess flap of skin that hangs over your penis. It has two important functions.

First, it protects the glans penis, the sensitive structure at the penis head. Second, the foreskin – which is sexually sensitive – allows the semen to be ejaculated quickly. In the dangerous world of our ancestors, they needed to be able to ejaculate before they were attacked by a beast or some other threat.

In addition to its protective and stimulatory functions, the foreskin also has a 'sliding' capacity in a partner who isn't sufficiently moist. Just as the Ancient Egyptians were able to transport heavy boulders on wooden rollers, the penis is able to 'roll' inside and penetrate the vagina thanks to its foreskin. Our distant ancestors made the most of this, because in an environment teeming with hungry predators there was little time for foreplay.

The foreskin has a bigger surface area than most people think. If you open it out completely, it is about the size of a postcard. That piece of skin is covered in sensory nerves with special nerve endings. These receive the sensory signals and send them to the brain, in turn triggering orgasm and ejaculation.

In 2013, our team in Ghent published a large study showing that the sensitivity of the foreskin plays an important role during sexual contact. So is sex with the foreskin better than without? The study didn't say. However, if the foreskin is still intact, it makes a considerable contribution to the sensations experienced. It is a question of a culmination of sensitivity: the glans penis of uncircumcised men is more sensitive in the first place; then add to that the sensitivity of the foreskin.

In any event, the glans penis of circumcised men is less sensitive than the glans penis of uncircumcised men. This is because the mucous membrane (the red covering) of the glans penis on circumcised men thickens slightly and so the nerve endings are located deeper in the mucous membrane. Circumcised men no longer experience the sensitivity of the foreskin, but that doesn't mean circumcised men can't have good sex. And some uncircumcised men experience too much sensitivity, so even their sex life isn't entirely carefree.

The sacrifice of the foreskin

At some point, someone must have been the first ever person to think about picking up a knife and cutting off their foreskin. Unfortunately, we will never know who that was. We can't even name one civilization as the inventor of circumcision. Quite separately from each other, human civilizations started circumcising men in what is now the Middle East, Australia and Polynesia, as did the Aztecs and the Mayas in what we now call Latin America.

We know that humans have been doing away with the protective flap of skin around the glans penis for a very long time. The oldest known illustration of a circumcision comes from Ancient Egypt and dates back as far as 5,000 years ago.

The practice took off and is still performed today. The World Health Organization estimates that 30 per cent of men are circumcised. That means 665 million exposed penis heads. This figure dates from 2007, and the world's population has since grown.

You may wonder what drove the first circumcised men to have their foreskin removed, long before any kind of anaesthesia. The penis is a precious and sensitive organ. Most men try to keep sharp objects well away from it.

However, there is some logic behind circumcision. One location where circumcision came about was in north-east Africa: the desert region. When uncircumcised men went to war, a combination of smegma, dust, sand and lack of water made the foreskin become inflamed. You can be as tough and strong a warrior as you like, but if your penis is inflamed you're good for nothing on the battlefield.

Historical sources suggest that a quarter of soldiers from this time fell sick from foreskin problems.

Historical sources suggest that a quarter of soldiers from this time, around 2500 BC, fell sick from foreskin problems. They couldn't urinate, they were in pain and they felt weak. This won't win any battles, so man must have reasoned at some point in time, 'If we take that flap of skin away, the problem is solved.' If, as a warrior, you saw the pain and discomfort of your fellow warriors, you would be quickly persuaded to offer up your foreskin. Circumcision therefore began as a practical procedure, a way of keeping soldiers healthy in an environment where they couldn't wash. This then reinforced the warrior's conviction that he was unbeatably strong if he was circumcised without anaesthesia and without letting out any cries of pain.

The custom was first only practised by warriors, but later it was practised on everyone. In any event, there wasn't a clear divide between citizens and soldiers; that distinction is a recent invention. The rulers had to 'sell' circumcision to ordinary people and you didn't do that by saying it was better for fighting wars. Religious reasons were far more effective.

So the practical custom of circumcision took on a religious connotation and then it acquired an *enigmatic* meaning. Ancient Egyptians offered their foreskin to Ra, the sun god, ignorant of the fact that sacrifice came in most handy when the Pharaoh was going to war. Later, the practice was taken on in various ways by other peoples from the region, for example the Jews and, later still, Arab Muslims.

The boundary between religion and ritual is very thin. In Judaism, circumcision is seen as a religious rite that determines who belongs to the Jewish people. Circumcision strictly takes place on the seventh day after birth.

Islam isn't as strict in determining when circumcision should take place. Instead, it tends to be a ritual somewhat like the Christian practice of first communion. It is a rite of passage.

In many African communities too, circumcision is considered a ritual to mark the transition from boy to man – or at least from child to adolescent. To make the transition physically apparent, circumcision was introduced – particularly in boys, but often in girls as well. In these communities, circumcision allowed a man to become sexually active. On the other hand, female circumcision is above all a manifestation of sexual repression, a way to deny women sexual pleasure.

In Africa, it's impossible to draw a line to show which groups circumcise and which groups don't. These customs are often far older than the advent of Christianity or Islam. There isn't even any uniformity within countries themselves. In the Congo, some groups do, some don't. In South Africa, men have for the most part been getting circumcised since the AIDS epidemic. A circumcised penis has a slightly less chance of contracting the HIV virus, but unfortunately circumcised men all too often think they are fully protected. This makes their risk of infection even greater, because they believe a condom isn't necessary.

The situation in the US is a different story altogether. Circumcision became popular there because of Puritanism. In the nineteenth century, John Harvey Kellogg – a medical doctor and the inventor of cornflakes – promoted circumcision as a way to stop boys from masturbating. The more unpleasant the circumcision, the better, reasoned Kellogg:

> *'The operation should be performed by a surgeon without administering an anesthetic, as the brief pain attending the operation will have a salutary effect upon the mind, especially if it be connected with the idea of punishment, as it may well be in some cases.'*

The aim of circumcision was explicitly to take pleasure away, which made the practice a form of organised child abuse. They still haven't completely removed the practice in the US. I recently acquired the book *Diseases Caused by Masturbation*, by the Swiss physician Samuel-Auguste Tissot. The book was written in 1760 and documents Tissot's view that semen is an 'essential oil' and 'stimulus' that, when lost from the body in great amounts, would cause 'a perceptible reduction of strength, of memory and even of reason; blurred vision, all the nervous disorders, all types of gout and rheumatism, weakening of the organs of generation, blood in the urine, disturbance of the appetite, headaches and a great number of other disorders.' Some people still consider Tissot's nonsense to be true.

If you look at the reality, you see that circumcised boys are still perfectly capable of masturbating, especially if they use lubricant. Lubricant is a perfectly normal item of use in the US. People buy it without any embarrassment and keep it on their bedside table. By contrast, in many Western European countries lubricant gets hidden away, both in the shop and in the bedroom.

Given that the main reason to circumcise boys isn't valid, advocates of circumcision come up with other reasons to remove the foreskin. A popular explanation is that circumcised men suffer from fewer urinary tract infections. That is correct, but concerns an extremely small group of men – namely those with a congenital disorder of the urinary tract, a condition that affects only 1 per cent of men.

Another reason cited by advocates is that circumcision reduces the risk of penile cancer. Penile cancer is a terrible thing, but this type of cancer is extremely rare. You can prove almost anything with statistics but the statistics in this case are really very weak. The number of lives you'd save does not outweigh the number of complications you cause. One per cent of circumcisions entail complications, which is more than the incidence of penile cancer. This makes the benefit of circumcision negligible.

... circumcised boys are still perfectly capable of masturbating, especially if they use lubricant. Lubricant is a perfectly normal item of use in the US.

Cervical cancer is another argument in favour of circumcision. Yes, it has been shown that cervical cancer is less common in Jewish women than in populations where men are usually not circumcised. Circumcised men appear to be less frequent carriers of the virus that causes cervical cancer – the human papilloma virus. But here too, the argument for general circumcision is far too weak. Circumcising the entire male population is not a sensible measure for reducing cervical cancer – vaccination against the virus is far more effective. You can prevent the majority of these cancers without having to remove the foreskin.

Advocates grapple somewhat between fact and fiction in their defence of circumcision. They face more and more resistance from progressive activists who argue for the practice to be banned altogether, especially in children who cannot give consent for such an intervention taking place on their penis.

The foreskin has become a symbol over which two camps are fiercely fighting.

A symbolic piece of skin

In the Old Testament, God gets straight to the point when he says to Abraham:

> *'This is my covenant which you shall keep, between me and you,*
> *and also with your offspring after you: Every male among you shall*
> *be circumcised. And you shall circumcise the flesh of your foreskin,*
> *and it shall be a sign of the covenant between me and you.'*

Such was the Word of God. Abraham, along with his offspring, had to sacrifice his foreskin – a sign of impurity – for the sake of Yahweh.

Imagine a sect nowadays saying, 'We're going to cut off a piece of you as an offering to God. Refusing is blasphemy.' The world would be turned upside down and it just wouldn't be possible any more.

The ritual of circumcision relies on a very long history and it was transformed from a practical custom into a religious symbol. It takes more than a few rational arguments to put something like that aside. It is very difficult to correct.

In the debate on circumcision, hypocrisy unfortunately all too often prevails. The World Health Organization views genital 'normalising' surgery on children as torture. This (extreme) viewpoint ensures that we no longer operate on children's genitals just like that, but the hypocrisy is that circumcision falls outside the definition of torture. It is viewed as only a small change. That might be so in some people's eyes, but circumcision actually remains a significant change.

The ban on genital surgery in children is all about the lack of consent, the balance between human rights and what is medically or culturally desirable. I'm not against circumcision personally, but I do think it's best to wait until a boy can decide for himself whether to be circumcised.

When a couple from Turkey came to see me with their young son, I said to them what I would always say to any parents asking for their child to be circumcised: 'I would prefer to wait until your son can decide for himself.' I notice in these cases that it's often not the parents who are desperate to get their son circumcised, but rather the pressure is coming from the grandparents.

I sympathise with people who are opposed to non-medical circumcision. It would be good if, in time, circumcisions would only happen with the subject's consent. But there is no point in forcing such things by law. You can only undo such customs by adequately convincing people over a long period of time.

In Germany, a boy took legal action against his parents for having him circumcised against his will. He won the case, albeit to the great dissatisfaction of religious minorities.

In Belgium, there is a lot of controversy surrounding health insurance reimbursements of circumcisions that aren't carried out for medical reasons. Opponents argue, 'A first communion isn't reimbursed, so why should circumcision be?'

We need to lead the debate, but we can't force it. We can't just remove circumcision from the list of reimbursed procedures without an alternative. We need to be very careful here, because otherwise circumcision will become clandestine and be carried out by people with no medical training. Or people will travel to countries where circumcision is less safe. Then we run the risk that young boys will be maimed anyway.

There is, however, an alternative and safety net in the Netherlands. People there can pay 300 euros for the procedure in an outpatient clinic. The system works.

In the US, the number of circumcisions performed on young boys is declining, it is now around the 50 per cent mark. The increasing awareness can also be seen in other statistics: for example, on pornographic websites, the search term 'uncut dick' is a lot more popular than the cut version.

Aside from religion, adults who consent to being circumcised have thousands of arguments for doing so. For example, to increase pleasure or improve the appearance.

I'm circumcised myself and that was my own choice. I was 24 and my boyfriend at the time was already circumcised. We talked about it for a long time and in the end I decided I would do it too. I've never regretted my decision. The most important thing, however, was that it was a *conscious* decision. I – and nobody else – was deciding about my foreskin.

If people are circumcised when they are old enough to make an informed decision, I have no problem with that. A Muslim who is circumcised later in life? Great idea!

Oops, there's been an accident

Circumcised men can sometimes feel pain in the underside of their penis during sex. Our own study confirmed this. The scar is located on the underside of the penis, so friction can cause an unpleasant sensation. After all, the entire complex of foreskin and penis skin works something like a sliding mechanism, and when it malfunctions, it can hurt.

When urologists circumcise a penis, it is usually for medical reasons. We take away what's not right and try to exclude complications as far as possible.

Fifteen per cent of men in Belgium are circumcised. If circumcisions were only performed for medical reasons, this figure would be just half a per cent or less.

The medical reasons to remove the foreskin, or a piece of it, are various. It could, for example, be necessary in men with a very long foreskin. Some diseases cause a narrowing of the foreskin, resulting in a thickening of the skin. The skin can also become cracked and scarred, causing discomfort or even pain during penetration. If a melanoma appears on the foreskin, we remove it. Removing the foreskin can also reduce excessive smegma production.

The decreased sensitivity after a circumcision isn't necessarily a bad thing. The more sensitive your penis, the easier you orgasm, but who wants to climax as quickly as possible per se? Sex isn't a race against the clock now that our homes protect us from hungry animals and curious onlookers. Circumcision can therefore bring solace to men who ejaculate prematurely, especially in combination with numbing lubricants. I always recommend trying numbing ointment first before sacrificing your foreskin.

... on pornographic websites, the search term 'uncut dick' is a lot more popular than the cut version.

In some men, premature ejaculation has nothing to do with penetration. They orgasm without anyone coming near their penis, just thinking about sex can be enough. Circumcision is pointless in these men. They can keep their foreskin and should seek a completely different treatment involving psychotherapy.

Outside the medical world, there are many different ways to perform circumcision. You could produce a catalogue. Variations include high, mid or low, loose or tight. You can keep the inner foreskin, fold it back and place it around the penis – this is called a 'high & tight circumcision'. Some retain more of the penis skin, meaning the flaccid penis has a bit of skin around the head, protecting it somewhat.

Every religion does it differently and there are even different practices within one religion. Some use clamps to kill off the foreskin, others use clamps to fuse the wound. Some stitch the wound, others bandage it and let it heal on its own.

A ritual circumcisor builds up a kind of professionalism after years of experience, but they are never truly authorised to cut the human body. Complications occur in 1 per cent of all circumcisions – but fortunately they are not all serious. If the remaining foreskin doesn't heal well, you will get some nasty scarring. Men who are circumcised too tight can suffer from painful erections. Worse still, I regularly see boys who are missing a bit of their glans. I even know boys who are missing a large part of their penis because of a circumcision carried out too enthusiastically.

Those are real dramas. The sexual future of such boys is heavily compromised: they have lost nearly all sensitive parts of their penis. I and my team developed a technique for making the penis look a bit more normal after such accidents. We enhance the erectile tissue to give the boy an extra centimetre in length and use the pink mucosa from the mouth to cover the tip of the penis, giving it a normal appearance again. The limitation of this method, however, is that we can't bring the sensitivity back, or at least not the sensitivity of a normal penis. You'll never have a perfect penis again after such an accident.

Boys who lose the most sensitive part of their penis often have problems with sexuality. They are sexually disabled. Having a small penis is nothing compared with having a penis that's lost its sensitivity. That can happen in circumcision or if a birth defect isn't treated properly. Such a thing is a personal tragedy.

We can do a lot these days. With phalloplasty, we try to find the nerve of the penis so that we can recover a bit of sensitivity. In boys with spina bifida, we connect the nerve in the penis to the nerve in the groin to enable sensation in the penis. But, as I said, the sensitivity that you lose if a circumcision goes wrong can never be restored.

All you can hope is that the remaining sensitivity in the penis and scrotum is enough to set the mechanism of orgasm and ejaculation in motion. Fortunately, our brains are extremely flexible and they can re-programme sensory signals with a bit of practice, making orgasm possible in such circumstances.

Reversing a circumcision, however, is impossible – whether successful or not. It is a question I'm asked more and more often and I always have to disappoint. The Ancient Greeks came up with a solution though. Physicians detached the skin at the base of the penis, slid it up and thus covered the glans. Scar tissue then grew on the exposed shaft. In a more recent version, a flap of skin was put over the wound, but this method was extremely ugly too. The practice is no longer practised anywhere, and a good job too. A covered glans can't justify the rest of your penis being mutilated.

What you do see nowadays are all kinds of gadgets to stretch the remaining foreskin. Some even hang weights on theirs. It works, but only for as long as you do it. If you keep it up for a very long time, until you reach the age where your skin loses its elasticity anyway, you might notice a permanent – albeit small – difference. You won't get a completely new foreskin though – not for the time being at least. With modern technology, we might be able to grow tissue from someone's own stem cells and sculpt it into the desired shape. That opens up possibilities of conjuring up a foreskin from a 3D printer. But such an invention is still far off, and even if the technology worked, organs like the liver and kidneys would have priority. A foreskin isn't so essential to survival.

Concerned mothers

Many parents see the doctor because they are concerned about their son's foreskin. But their concerns aren't always good for boys. Some parents think they need to pull the foreskin back heavily, and that can be traumatising. This concern usually doesn't have any foundation: the foreskin only needs to roll completely past the crown of the glans when the boy is sexually active.

Is the foreskin sticking to the glans? Or is the foreskin tight but with no signs of disease? It can't do a young boy any harm – so let's not create problems where there aren't any. These adhesions and physiological narrowings are normal – they occur in almost half of boys who haven't yet reached puberty. We sometimes refer to this as the virginity of boys.

There are no bacteria under the adhesion, or only 'good' bacteria, which are part of the penis's normal microbiome. An adhered foreskin isn't dirty and it doesn't need washing per se. It is a myth that you need to be able to retract the foreskin of a young boy, a myth we need to put to rest as soon as possible. When puberty comes, the adhesions resolve on their own, if need be with the help of night-time erections or masturbation.

Sometimes smegma builds up under the adhesion, causing inflammation. In that case, we intervene by rubbing anaesthetic ointment on the foreskin, leaving it to work for 30 minutes and then detaching the adhesion. It is completely painless. When the physiological narrowing of the foreskin looks like it's going to cause problems, our solution is to apply cortisone ointment for a few weeks. This helps 90 per cent of patients.

There are too many myths around about the foreskin. So much folklore is based on customs that have no factual, medical or scientific basis. One must also be wary of doctors recommending circumcisions when they work in healthcare systems that financially reward doctors for the number of services performed.

In essence though, it's simple: you should concern yourself as little as possible with the foreskin unless a doctor says something is seriously wrong, and in cases like this you should ask about non-surgical solutions as well. Ninety-nine per cent of boys have a perfectly normal foreskin though. Leave it be.

Looking after your foreskin

The foreskin isn't unhygienic. But that doesn't mean that it is sterile. There is such a thing as the penile microbiome: a colony of bacteria who have set up home underneath the foreskin.

Bacteria are a living part of every human being – on average, we carry around two kilograms of bacteria on us – and different colonies are found in different parts of the body. This means the microbiome of the mouth is different to that of the skin, the intestine or the vagina, etc. There is a colony of different bacteria under the foreskin of an uncircumcised man too.

The bacterial composition determines the health of that moist environment found under the foreskin, where the sebaceous secretion called smegma is produced. If the bacterial balance is disturbed, this can cause problems. Minor problems include a bad smell or excessive smegma production; more serious is inflammation of the foreskin.

If you look after your foreskin with water and soap (preferably pH-neutral or slightly acidic) and rinse it well, there is no reason why your penis should be less hygienic than one without a foreskin. The smell of fresh smegma can even have a stimulating effect during sex.

If you don't look after your foreskin though, it will get dirty. There are myths out there that you mustn't use soap at all. You can, but don't use too much and rinse the residue off. Definitely don't use antibacterial soap, because otherwise you might disturb the bacterial balance and cause inflammation.

Fortunately, the hygiene of European penises is good overall.

How sexual activity affects the microbiome under the foreskin isn't entirely clear. Obviously, there is an exchange of bacteria in the case of vaginal sex. Part of the vaginal microbiome finds a new place to live under the foreskin, just as some of the microbiome of the mouth relocates during oral sex. Unprotected anal sex gives the microbiome of the rectum a night on the town.

To date, there have been no good quality scientific studies about these movements of bacteria, but we assume that the exchange of healthy colonies doesn't cause any problems. However, if a microbiome becomes imbalanced, it can affect other microbiomes. Therefore, bacterial vaginosis is a common bacterial infection where the proliferation of one type of bacteria disturbs the pH of the vagina. The condition can affect the microbiome under the foreskin, but men don't usually get any symptoms.

Sexually transmitted infections can also find a home under the foreskin, but in such cases a disturbance of the penile microbiome is the least of your worries.

The dreaded zip

When you take a pee, what do you do with your foreskin: pull it back or not? In principle, you don't have to do anything. Urine is a sterile fluid and therefore isn't dirty. It's also not true that you'll pee under your foreskin if you don't pull it back. Thanks to a very small muscle, the foreskin stays nice and close to the glans, it even presses against it slightly. During urination, the stream of urine chooses the shortest route and that's outwards, through the opening in the foreskin, without getting the entire penis head wet. But although you don't have to pull your foreskin back when you urinate, you can if you want to. Whichever you do, it won't do any harm.

Like so many physical body characteristics, there are huge variations in the size of every man's foreskin. In exceptional cases, when some men have a very long foreskin, it is possible to get a build-up of urine while urinating. These men do find it better if they pull their foreskin back. Others might also find they can control the urine stream better with their foreskin pulled back.

What you do with your foreskin *after* urinating is perhaps a lot more important than what you do with it during. Circumcised men have one advantage here: their foreskin will never get trapped in their trouser zip. They are spared that worry.

What do you do if the nightmare becomes reality and you want to pass out from the pain? Certainly don't undo the zip again, or you'll feel the unbearable pain of the zip a second time. That much punishment is never necessary!

The best thing to do is cut out the zip with a pair of cutters, so you can carefully pull the teeth apart. Or cut the zip underneath the bit where your foreskin is caught and pull the zip teeth apart in the same way.

If you're feeling resistant to damaging the zip, tell yourself the trousers will wear out eventually anyway. Ideally, you want to keep your foreskin for life.

4

The erection

One organ, two forms

The penis can take two different forms. In flaccid state, the penis is an innocent attachment to the male body. A male can urinate with it – and that's all. A flaccid penis has no other purpose than that.

For a long time, there were no sexual connotations attached to a flaccid penis. Up until the nineteenth century, swimming naked was common and no-one paid any attention to a penis if it was in the vicinity of a lake – so long as it stayed flaccid.

In the (in many ways puritanical) United States, it was even *compulsory* to swim naked in YMCA swimming baths, as bacteria found their way all too easily into the cotton swimwear of the time. Once women were allowed to go to the YMCA, they had to wear a bathing suit for moral reasons. You therefore see photos of stark-naked men next to (reasonably) demurely clothed women – an image that would surprise us these days. Only in the 1970s, when synthetic bathing suits made an appearance and chlorine was used on a large scale in swimming pools, did men get the right to protect their modesty.

The flaccid penis disappeared from view. You barely ever see them now in public and they only very rarely appear in the media, usually in a medical context. Only in theatres is a naked penis considered artistic tradition; they are all but absent in the cinema. Surely now that social media determines our image culture, the penis will be banished to the corners of the internet where only adults can go.

As flaccid penises vanished from public life, it meant that the penis was now most commonly seen in public as erect (through pornography). In this stiff, erect form, the penis is no longer an innocent attachment. It stands up proudly. Swollen veins meander up the hard shaft. The foreskin rolls back revealing a gleaming glans that points up towards the sky. In this form, the penis only has one goal. Sex.

Never has more pornography been produced than today and yet, at the same time, the phallus has disappeared more than ever from the public eye.

Phalluses have been the symbol of male strength and fertility for thousands of years. Pre-historic cave paintings depict hunters with erections and countless sculptures represent men with a prominent erect penis. Often, there isn't even a man attached to the phallus, as though the erection is separate from its owner. Phalluses were part of public life all over the world, they decorated temples and homes. Fertility was, after all, a valuable asset.

When the erection appeared in drawings or paintings, the wearer's face was full of lust. The other figures in the painting weren't doing everyday tasks like spinning yarn or making furniture: everyone surrendered to his or her sexual urge.

Over time, sex became a taboo. You had to reproduce, but getting pleasure from it was morally pernicious. Erotic images disappeared into the private sphere, and thus the pornography market emerged. Even in the early days of photography in the nineteenth century, men were flaunting their erections in front of the lens, and not just for decorative or scientific purposes. Their aim was to make money with erotic pictures, which were coveted precisely because of their clandestine nature.

Never has more pornography been produced than today and yet, at the same time, the phallus has disappeared more than ever from the public eye. You don't see any erections in the newspapers. If an article reports on an erection, it is usually medical news or reports of improper behaviour. Sometimes a too-public phallus causes controversy – such as in May 2018, when visitors of Middelheim Park in Antwerp, Belgium set their eyes on a sculpture of a man who was unapologetically pointing his erection towards the tree tops. They said the sculpture was offensive and unsuitable for a public place. The sculpture was moved to a hidden corner of the park, so that fewer people would be offended.

An erection is inextricably linked to sex and for many people an image of an erection is by definition pornographic and no longer art. This applies to the penis as a whole, even in its flaccid, innocent form.

The fact that the sexual connotation of the erection has now made its way to the flaccid penis as well isn't entirely illogical – it is one and the same organ after all. The stiff, erect alter ego has cast its shadow over its flaccid variant, which is now also under suspicion. Groups of people are always publishing naked calendars for a good cause, but never with penises in the frame – it has to stay honourable and even a flaccid penis is a step too far. This is because, in principle, any penis can suddenly stick its head up and change form.

The erect penis wasn't created to look nice or to seduce. The image of an erection won't automatically turn on heterosexual women. There's no consensus among women as to the erotic nature of the erection. While few heterosexual men are indifferent to female breasts, breasts don't even have a function during coitus.

The shape of the erection is purely functional. In an erect state, the penis is adapted to a very specific environment: the female vagina. Its only purpose is to penetrate and perform intercourse. There is no other organ with a more direct link to sex than the erect penis. The vagina is a coital organ too, but it also functions as a birth canal. An erection exists only for intercourse. It is precisely this multifunctional vagina that shaped the penis over millions of years into its current form.

Fossils of our human-like ancestors show that female hips adapted to the increasing head circumference of newborns. Early human species were becoming more and more intelligent, meaning their brain volume was increasing as well. The birth canal followed this trend and, through sexual selection, the penis grew too. Not only do we have a bigger penis than other apes, the shape is also more pronounced. All evidence suggests that the prominent penis crown also came about under the influence of the vagina.

We can therefore assume that the human erection has human intelligence to thank indirectly for its size and shape. But this explanation changes nothing of the way in which the penis is perceived. Endless discussions can be had on the appearance of the penis. Is it an attractive-looking organ or not? And is the penis most attractive when flaccid or erect?

Perhaps there are as many opinions about this as there are people. Penises also vary in shape, especially when erect, giving us further differences in opinion still. Does long look nicer than short; is wide more attractive than narrow? Then we have the penis head, the glans: how big should this be in relation to the rest of the penis, and is a pronounced corona (penis crown) preferable to a discreet ridge? Some glans are purple-red, others are deep red, and others have a more pinkish tinge: which is most attractive out of those?

Despite all doubts about aesthetic appearance, there *is* such a thing as an ideal proportion in terms of length in relation to width, and size of the glans in relation to the penis as a whole. When erect, the ideal proportion between length and circumference is 13.12 centimetres versus 11.66 centimetres respectively (1:12 if you calculate the ratio). If the measurements deviate significantly from the ideal, the penis will stand out in the eyes of the average person; for example a short and wide or long and narrow penis.

Porn actress Stormy Daniels was allegedly astonished by what she saw between the legs of Donald Trump. She compared the presidential penis to the mushroom character from the video game *Mario Kart*. The description is certainly cute, but is a penis like that attractive too?

You can wonder at all the possible shapes and sizes, but the real wonder is how a flaccid organ can suddenly get hard and erect. The mechanism behind it is very simple nonetheless.

A mechanical swelling

I can't stand the terms 'blood penis' and 'meat penis'. Everyone actually has a blood penis, no-one has meat in theirs. The term 'blood penis' is used to refer to a penis that is small when flaccid but grows very big when erect. A 'meat penis' is supposed to be just as long when flaccid as when erect.

Unfortunately for those who believe this, it doesn't work like that.

The only thing that can explain the difference between a so-called blood and meat penis is the subcutaneous dartos muscle, as we saw earlier. This is more active in some men and so it draws the flaccid penis inwards. Other men have a lazy dartos muscle, so their number hangs down prominently in a flaccid state. The two terms are incorrect because it is precisely the blood penis that has most muscle.

Humans don't have a penis bone either, unlike other apes such as the gorilla and chimpanzee. In many animals, the presence of a penis bone is associated with the duration of sexual penetration. Walruses, for example, specialise in prolonged copulation and have a penis bone measuring up to 60 centimetres, the longest example in the animal kingdom.

The penis bone has disappeared from humans by natural selection; human erections come about purely via hydraulics. There is some logic behind this: as the head circumference of newborns grew, so did the penis, but sex for prehistoric humans had to take place as quickly as possible. Hydraulics offer the advantage of allowing the penis to grow to a considerable size but letting the erection disappear again in the blink of an eye.

The rapid change in shape is the exclusive feature of a penis; no other organ can become harder and longer in such a short period of time. This unique mechanism is based on the blood supply to the three expandable tubes of erectile tissue. If you were to cut a penis through the middle, you would see these three columns very clearly. There are the two corpora cavernosa, which point the erection upwards. The third column is the corpus spongiosum, through which the urethra passes.

The penis bone has disappeared from humans by natural selection; human erections come about purely via hydraulics.

At rest, an equal amount of blood flows into and out of the corpora. During an erection, the blood supply increases and the outflow is closed off. This means more blood goes in than out, and the penis swells and becomes erect. Thanks to the specific structure of the corpora, they swell to a certain volume and then come up against pressure. The penis is not only swollen, it feels hard too.

It's the same system as with tyres on a bike. If you pump up the inner tube, the volume increases, but without the outer tyre the inner tube would keep swelling until it blows. The outer tyre provides counter-pressure. It's exactly the same principle in the penis. Blood collects in the inner tube and the tunica albuginea (the fibrous envelope of the corpora) acts like an outer tyre. Without this counter-pressure, your penis would rupture or never reach its desired hardness.

The corpus spongiosum also becomes hard, but not as hard as the two corpora cavernosa. The glans is attached to this tissue, so although it swells during an erection, it doesn't get too hard.

I once saw a patient with a very specific complaint, 'My glans doesn't get hard enough,' he complained.

That's how it should be. The corpus spongiosum mustn't be too hard or the sperm won't be able to pass through the urethra; the urethra would be pressed shut.

The glans penis

The erect penis is not just an even, fleshy shaft. It has a characteristic crown, which shimmers when erect: the glans or head of the penis. The medical term *glans penis* comes from the Latin for 'acorn' of the penis. The comparison to the fruit of the oak is down to the archetypal crown that runs around it: the corona of glans penis.

Where does the corona of glans penis come from? No-one can answer that question with certainty, but there are theories to explain the path that evolution took.

We have already seen that the reason why humans have the biggest penis is down to the size of the vagina, which adapted to the larger head of a human baby. The corona of glans penis also adapted to the vagina, but we still don't know what its function is.

The relatively thick boundary of the glans increases the suction effect of the penis. Some think that its wider dimension helps remove the sperm of any predecessors from the vagina, so that the man's own sperm has less competition. This partially explains why the top of the penis looks a bit like a toilet plunger.

Another more likely explanation is to do with the hostile environment of the vagina itself. A healthy vagina has a low pH level and sperm cells are sentenced to death in that acidic environment if they don't quickly make their way towards the womb and fallopian tubes. Sperm that's left behind might not be competition any more, but it can block the way for a new army of sperm cells.

The corona doesn't so much remove competing sperm, but rather the hostile vaginal fluids that attack the sperm cells. Thanks to its specific shape, the glans drives the vaginal fluid to the entrance of the vagina, leaving the coast clear for the sperm cells to land deep within the vagina.

The theories don't stop there. The mucous membrane in the vagina and the Bartholin's glands (glands at the entrance of the vagina) produce vaginal discharge, which contains a range of substances. The acidity of this discharge protects the vagina from germs, but the discharge also contains neuropeptides. These are substances with which nerve cells communicate and which also function like hormones. The assumption is that these substances collect in the groove (sulcus) under the corona and they are then absorbed by the mucous membrane of the foreskin. Some hypotheses suggest that the female hormones arouse a feeling of connection in the man. In that sense, sexual intercourse is a form of communication older than spoken language. Whether the theory will survive thorough scientific research remains to be seen, but it is a nice thought all the same.

Humans aren't the only species with a wide glans. The glans is especially wide in animals whose copulation lasts a long time. In some animals, the glans is more club-shaped to keep the penis firmly in place. At the same time, a wide glans ensures the sperm doesn't trickle out and travels quickly to the egg. An example of this is a horse.

With mating dogs, the penis can sometimes get stuck in the vagina. This is known as a *penis captivus,* or a trapped penis. Persistent rumours exist of this happening in humans, but I've never had a patient report such a thing to me. I don't know what remedy vets use to solve the problem. Perhaps a bucket of cold water will do the trick to kill the erection with a fight-or-flight response.

Because copulation is briefer in hominids (great apes, gorillas, humans etc), the glans doesn't have to hold the penis in place so much. The cone shape of the glans makes it easier for the penis to penetrate the vagina and its wide corona helps prevent the penis from slipping out, but that's not the most important function. Indeed, a woman's clitoris also has a rim, but the external part of the clitoris is too short to penetrate anything. The clitoris only has one purpose: to trigger an orgasm. And that's precisely where we should be looking for an explanation of the wide base of the glans, because this is where the largest concentration of nerve endings are found.

The fact that the widest part of the penis is also the most sensitive ensures the man can quickly climax.

The corona of glans penis is the widest structure of the penis and so, during penetration, it is the part that rubs most against the vaginal wall. The corona thus ensures maximum stimulation, both in the vagina and for the man himself. The fact that the widest part of the penis is also the most sensitive ensures the man can quickly climax. Again, that came in most handy in pre-historic times, when a speedy ejaculation was desirable to avoid ending up in the jaws of a hungry animal.

The glans gets back-up here from the frenulum, the elastic band of tissue that connects the glans to the foreskin. The frenulum holds a high concentration of sensory nerves too. During sexual stimulation, whether by penetration or masturbation, the frenulum comes repeatedly under tension. This increases the sensation in uncircumcised men in particular.

The corona can sometimes have small bumps around it, called pearly penile papules, which are usually found in rows. These stand out more in some men than others. They're nothing to worry about, they aren't warts that you've contracted from unprotected sex. We assume that these papules bring about extra stimulation. Cats even have penile spines (which serve both directions), and as a castrated cat loses these projections we can assume that the penile papules have a sexual intention.

I sometimes see patients who are worried about their pearly penile papules or don't like the look of them. We can remove these protuberances with a laser beam, but then nerve endings will undoubtedly come under fire too. You always have to ask if it's really worth risking a piece of your sensitivity for the sake of a slightly better appearance.

During an erection, the mucous membrane of the glans becomes taut. This is often darker than the rest of the penis. Many mothers come to me concerned that their child's glans is blue. This is quite normal. The mucous membrane of the glans is relatively thin in children, so the slow flow of blood gives it a dark blue appearance. You can compare it to the blue veins on the back of your hand.

You get a variety of shades when it comes to colour of the glans in adults too. Dark-red, purple, pink: they are all normal. The glans is also red or reddish in men with a darker skin tone, it's just slightly more pigmented.

The wayward erection

Getting the onset of an erection on a nudist beach or in a sauna is embarrassing. But science offers a small bit of consolation: there's nothing you can do about it. You have no say at all in your erection. The autonomic nervous system decides for you when your manhood is going to get stiff.

Moving your arm or legs is something you do consciously using the somatic (or voluntary) nervous system. The autonomic (involuntary) nervous system controls the heart, intestines, bladder filling, and also the erection. Just as you can't make your heart stop, nor can you summon an erection on cue – or make it disappear.

The autonomic nervous system has two components: the parasympathetic and sympathetic nervous systems. The sympathetic nervous system prepares the body for the flight-or-fight response and accelerates the body. The parasympathetic nervous system brings the body to rest.

Healthy men get an erection between six and eight times a night, and usually don't even notice it.

The penis is the exception. It is the parasympathetic nervous system that brings about an erection, whereas the flight-or-fight response makes the penis go limp – for example, if a policeman turns up when two people are having sex in the bushes.

The parasympathetic nervous system doesn't need the brain in order to do its work. Look at patients with a serious spinal cord injury: not a single signal reaches the lower body from the head and yet local stimuli can trigger an erection, although they don't feel it because sensations take place in the head.

You can't voluntarily decide to get an erection, but you can trigger an erection by consciously thinking erotic thoughts. An erection might also appear because you feel like having sex. Arousing images or smells can also trigger an erection. Hormones play a role in this: desire for sex – the famous libido – is heavily influenced by sex hormones.

The parasympathetic nervous system means a man can get an erection when he doesn't even fancy sex. Stimuli on the penis can even cause an erection when you categorically don't feel like sex. For boys and men who fall victim to unwanted intimacies, this mechanism, on top of the trauma, can instil a feeling of guilt: *'I got an erection, so I must have wanted it...'*

Far more innocent are night-time erections. Healthy men get an erection between six and eight times a night, and usually don't even notice it. You don't think about sex while you sleep – unless you're having an erotic dream – and your penis still gets hard. Once again, it's the parasympathetic nervous system that's responsible for this. Your penis responds to direct stimuli from your pyjamas, the bedclothes, or your bed partner's body. Or the parasympathetic nervous system simply activates itself, without any external stimuli at all.

Every man is familiar with the morning erection, the erection you wake up with. That is actually the last night-time erection. Because your bladder is full, an additional nerve signal is sent to the penis, making the erection a bit more constant. The testosterone level is also at its highest in the morning. The male hormone level fluctuates during the 24-hour period of the day, and we don't know exactly why it peaks on waking up. Evolution gives us one possible explanation: if you wake up in the morning, it means you have survived the night and you are probably in a safe location. You can make the most of this by having a go at reproducing. Whatever the reason, the additional peak in hormone levels makes morning erections an indisputable fact.

So what is the point in having a sequence of night-time erections? After all, you don't have sex while you sleep. That's true, but night-time erections maintain the mechanism. If a car sits unused for too long during the winter months, it might get a flat battery just when you need it most. It's the same with the penis: if you only get an erection when you need it for sex, the mechanism might fail just when you want it to work.

There are people who claim that night-time erections supply extra oxygen to the penis and that this oxygenation therapy is good for your health. That may be so, but I'd say such a thing is probably more incidental.

Night-time erections tell us something about the health of your circulatory system. If you're not getting erections at night any more, it's time to see a cardiologist. In the past, we used the postage stamp test to assess this. A man would secure a strip of postage stamps around his penis before going to sleep and if the strip was broken come the morning, he had had a night-time erection: a good sign. We no longer do that. Not because the test didn't work, but because postage stamps are now self-adhesive!

Night-time erections also maintain penis length. You can think of it like a form of stretching. Unfortunately, the cycle malfunctions in impotent men, so their penis often gets shorter. This is because without the night-time stretch the corpora have a tendency to shrink over time. The tissue of the tunica albuginea (which envelopes the erectile tissue) is fibrous tissue and the fibres tend to shorten when they are not stretched. So the night-time erections help to maintain the penile length. The shortening is not dramatic but it can be a few centimetres after several years.

Erectile dysfunction

The vast majority of erectile problems share the same symptom: the penis no longer gets erect and isn't hard enough to enable penetration.

A whole range of issues lead to that one, highly unfortunate, clinical picture. To begin with, the problem can be related to the nerves. A disease like diabetes damages the nerves, so sensory stimuli don't get through and you feel too little stimulation to get an erection.

The problem could also be to do with the blood supply, for example with atherosclerosis. Atherosclerosis is a disease where fatty deposits (plaque) clog up the arteries, in the same way as with high cholesterol. Because the erectile tissue mechanism needs blood, any blood vessel disorder can affect an erection. The blood vessels of the penis are even finer than the vessels that supply the heart. They are therefore quicker to get blocked. Smoking, diabetes and obesity do little to help penis stiffness.

Likewise, the blood supply may be perfectly fine, but there might be too much outflow, for example with a leaking blood vessel. If you have an erection but you can squeeze your penis until it becomes soft, that might be amusing to watch, but it *isn't* normal. You've almost certainly got a venous leak – a tear in a vessel causing loss of pressure.

This could be congenital or caused by a trauma. A typical case would be the connection between the erectile tissue and a vein under the penis skin. The blood then drains away in a manner that isn't intended.

Peyronie's disease can be caused by a trauma whereby the tunica albuginea (fibrous envelope of the erectile tissue) becomes so hard and damaged that blood drains away via an unorthodox exit. Most people with this disease have a bent erection, but some no longer get an erection at all.

If you can squeeze your penis until it becomes soft, that might be amusing to watch, but it *isn't* normal.

The majority of erectile dysfunctions are caused by a problem with blood supply, but sometimes the problem can be hormonal. If hormones don't sufficiently maintain the libido, erections become rarer, too.

You get your best quality erections from puberty through to your twenties. From a purely biological perspective, males are also most fertile as an adolescent and young adult. The need for hard, reliable erections is greatest at this age.

Nowadays, though, humans live a lot longer than is necessary to procreate. We also remain sexually active long after our optimal reproductive age. Because sex has been dissociated from reproduction, the pressure to get erections is even greater. If you stay healthy, you can in principle get normal erections up until your nineties. Unfortunately though, many people don't lead healthy lives so they become dependent on pills or other aids.

Ageing is detrimental to the erection on various levels. The reduced production of hormones decreases your libido, so in turn your penis needs more encouragement to get erect. The erection is one of the first casualties when age-related ailments make an appearance. The older you are, the greater the chance that you suffer from obesity, diabetes and atherosclerosis, known plaguers of the erection.

If you don't have any physical ailments and your hormone levels are normal, stress or uncertainty can play their part in making sure your penis doesn't get erect. In this case, the reason for your erection problems lies between your ears.

You get your best quality erections from puberty through to your twenties.

The typical psychogenic cause is anxiety. Anxiety is the biggest enemy of an erection. You can get rid of your hiccups by being startled, but this works for your erection too. Anyone ever caught masturbating by their mum will confirm it: your erection is gone in a flash.

A brief shock like that though isn't an erection problem. Rather, we are interested in chronic anxiety disorders. Someone with performance anxiety, for example, might have an unfortunate experience where he can't get hard, exacerbating his anxiety. Boys with a genital birth defect can be so scared of being laughed at that their erection simply bites the dust. Men who worry about their penis length, whether they have a legitimate concern or not, see their erection go up in smoke because their worry or anxiety is so great.

This is an effect of the sympathetic nervous system responsible for our flight-or-fight response. Anxiety releases adrenaline in the blood and makes our heart beat faster. The blood vessels that we don't need to survive constrict. Whether you fight or run away, your muscles need oxygen; all the blood flows to your muscles, leaving none spare for the erectile tissue in your penis. Your erection loses its hardness and your penis hangs its head. That's logical really: if you have to fight or run for your life, sex is the last thing on your mind. Even if you *know* that you don't have to 'fight or flight', the sympathetic nervous system still holds the reins.

Unless you are actually standing in front of a wild animal, fear is usually a bad advisor. I therefore tell adolescents with anxiety to take a low dose of an erection pill to give their self-confidence a boost so they can overcome their fear. That can temper the whims of the sympathetic nervous system.

Hard guarantees

In simple terms, an erection is a purely physical process: corpora cavernosa fill with blood and the harder they are pumped, the harder the erection.

In reality, chemistry plays a part too. In the sequence of chemical reactions that lead to an erection, one molecule plays a key role: nitric oxide, or 'NO' for chemists. This colourless gas is produced, among other things, by the burning of fossil fuel in cars and thermal power stations. Nitric oxide widens the blood vessels, allowing them to fill with blood and make the penis hard.

The pharmaceutical industry has utilised this principle to tackle erection problems. All pills that help maintain an erection ensure that nitric oxide is broken down more slowly. Previously, we had to administer injections in the penis to prevent the breakdown of nitric oxide locally; pills make life a lot easier.

When pills don't work any more, we put in a penile implant, giving your penis a new inner tube made from silicone.

The principle is simple: a water-filled balloon reservoir is put in your abdomen and this is connected to a pump in your scrotum. You then pump water from the reservoir in your abdomen to the new inner tubes in the erectile tissue, and your penis becomes hard and erect. The water is drained back to the low-pressure reservoir in your abdomen at the push of a button. It works very well.

With today's technological advancements and innovations, I'm sure it won't be long before we see automatic systems on the market that are operated by remote control. Can you imagine the arguments in the bedroom about whether to turn the erection on or off? And what if the remote control gets lost?

In the future we might use stem cells to repair erectile tissue. The inside of the erectile tissue is made of very special cells that get the nitric oxide factory working. Age-related ailments affect their work and you end up with softer erections. By implanting stem cells, we can repair the chemical factory in the tunica albuginea and get the system going again.

A far older and purely mechanical alternative to support the erection is the vacuum pump. A tube is placed over the penis and then all the air is sucked out of the tube. Some systems work manually, others offer the comfort of an electric motor. Its modus operandi is that the vacuum in the tube draws extra blood to the penis.

Once the penis is sufficiently filled and hard, you put a seal around the base of the penis. This prevents the extra blood from draining away. Remove the tube, and so long as the seal is still in place, you'll have a stiff penis. One disadvantage is that the penis is only stiff between the seal and the glans, whereas the erectile tissue runs far deeper in your body. This can make the penis sway to and fro, like a hard trunk on a soft base. That can look funny, but it means your penis needs manual support to achieve penetration.

Porn actors also use the vacuum pump, in addition to erection pills, to give their performance that *je ne sais quoi*. Such a device isn't actually suitable for this. And it doesn't really work on someone who has normal erections.

Men with Peyronie's disease sometimes benefit when they use a vacuum pump for 30 minutes a day. Peyronie's disease causes some of the erectile tissue structures to harden or too much scar tissue to form, making the erection bent. We try to soften the scars by regularly stretching the penis with a vacuum pump. Injections have also recently become available to soften the scars. That sometimes works, but for many patients with Peyronie's disease, an operation is the only guaranteed way of getting a straight penis back again.

Mr Persistence has a problem

An erection shouldn't last for ever. A prolonged erection is unhealthy, even. When an erection won't go away, you're talking about priapism.

The condition is named after Priapus, the Greek god of fertility. Frescoes in the Roman city of Pompeii depict him strutting his enormous penis. Priapus may have been the protector of the penis, but anyone who suffers from priapism is right to be concerned.

There are various causes of priapism. Sometimes it can be the side effect of certain medication, such as anti-depressants, or if a particular kind of medication works too well. Before the advent of the erection pill, men with erectile problems would see a urologist for an injection in their penis. This injection activates the erection, but it can also make the penis erect for an unsuitably long time. Some blood disorders can also cause priapism.

Your penis is likely to survive *high-flow* priapism, caused by an excessive inflow of blood. It is *low-flow* priapism, where the outflow of blood is impaired, that can be particularly harmful. This causes too little blood to circulate in the penis, meaning too little oxygen gets to the penis. If the erection lasts more than 24 hours, your penis will be irreparably damaged.

The effect is similar, if you like, to what would happen if you wrapped an elastic band around your thumb a few times. First, your thumb would become red and swollen, because the blood can't escape. If you didn't remove the elastic band, no new oxygen would get in and the local tissue would die. Your thumb would turn black.

Priapism won't make your penis turn black and fall off – that only happens in very extreme cases – but the entire chemical factory inside your penis is damaged. If you wait too long to see a doctor about priapism, you'll never be able to get a spontaneous erection again and the only help for you will be a penile implant. So forget your embarrassment and save your penis.

It's also important that your penis doesn't become a workaholic: after work it has to rest. A healthy body is prepared for this: the typical sex cycle involves arousal first, followed by the sexual activity itself and orgasm as the high point and end point. The cycle lasts a little longer still: after orgasm comes the refractory period. A short circuit makes the erection disappear, making it impossible to get a new erection for the next few minutes. This is the body's way of protecting itself against priapism and giving the penis a fresh shot of oxygen.

Some men would prefer not to have an erection that goes soft right after the first orgasm. And so we see inventions like the cock ring – a metal or rubber ring that you wear around your penis to slow down the flow of blood. This creates an artificial form of priapism.

It's not harmful in itself, but if you use a cock ring too often and for too long, it can cause damage. If you can't get the ring off, you have a serious problem – and just like with real priapism, you must seek medical help straight away. We regularly transport victims to the operating theatre to put our hard-core equipment to good use – fortunately our orthopaedists always have a sterile concrete cutter on hand. The patient doesn't have to watch – he's under general anaesthesia.

Although the penis was created to be able to get an erection, an erection is by definition a temporary occurrence. As soon as the penis has done its work, the structure must come down again. The penis must rest. After all, the real purpose of the penis isn't to get erections, but to deliver sperm.

5

Sperm

A sticky substance

Sperm, or semen, is a whitish fluid. All post-pubescent men, and also perhaps most women, know where it comes from: the penis during an orgasm.

It is a highly effective substance because, invisible to the naked eye, it contains millions of sperm cells.

Semen has a certain sticky consistency to it, termed 'viscous' by natural scientists. Its viscosity isn't down to chance; it is the result of evolution and serves a purpose. That purpose is to give the sperm cells as good a chance as possible of fertilising an egg.

The basic principle of reproduction is that the more partners a man has the more chance you have of successfully reproducing. But if a female has several partners, your chance of fertilising her egg becomes smaller. In some animals, therefore, the semen forms a resin-like plug in the vagina, blocking access to sperm cells of men that come after. This means they can walk away after sex and kill two birds with one stone: they don't end up the next meal of another animal and their sperm stays in place, without them having to keep competitors away from the female.

In humans, this shut-off function has disappeared – partner relationships have become more stable and promiscuity has to some extent decreased. However, semen still hasn't become a watery fluid. To prevent all the sperm from trickling out when a woman stands up after sex, it has to have a certain stickiness. The viscosity of human semen varies greatly, from runny to not runny at all. The variety is as great as the variety of men.

Semen comes out the penis with some force, albeit in limited volume. The average semen ejaculation has a volume of five millilitres, equivalent to one coffee spoon. The vast majority of men, namely 95 per cent, ejaculate between two and eight millilitres of semen. Anything between these values is completely normal. Any volumes bigger or smaller than this are produced by a very small minority, but they are not abnormal.

Porn actors always appear to ejaculate a lot more than eight millilitres – but please don't view the volumes in porn films as standard, because they are fake. It sometimes looks like these actors ejaculate litres of sperm, but these plentiful cumshots are the result of cunning montage.

Experts compare the smell of semen to chestnut blossom or the Chinese Callery pear tree.

The only way to increase the volume ejaculated is to wait a long time between ejaculations or be more sexually stimulated than normal – that's not the norm in the porn industry, because ejaculating is the daily routine. In order to ejaculate a sufficient volume, you must also be in good health and drink enough water – 1.5 to 2 litres a day.

The colour of semen starts off translucent white. After a few minutes it loses its white colour and becomes more fluid.

Experts compare the smell of semen to chestnut blossom or the Chinese Callery pear tree. There are very few people who think: *Mmm, that smells of chestnut blossom,* when they smell semen. Rather, it's the other way round. The first time you catch a scent of chestnut blossom, you think: *Hehe, that smells of sperm.*

People with a rich olfactory imagination think that semen tastes of almonds. The actual taste of semen is more unpleasant than that. It's not supposed to taste nice either, otherwise we'd eat it and that's not the aim. If semen tasted like honey, a lot more oral sex would take place and a lot fewer eggs would be fertilised. It would defeat the object of the exercise: to ensure reproduction. If online porn is anything to go by, there is enough ejaculating in faces and mouths as it is.

The fact that semen doesn't taste delicious doesn't mean it tastes repulsively bad. You can influence the taste of your ejaculate by what you do – or don't – eat, because the flavour of garlic or asparagus, for example, ends up in your semen. I once read somewhere – albeit from a source with little scientific evidence – that pineapple in particular made semen taste sweet.

The sperm factory

Testosterone is needed to make sperm cells, otherwise the testicles don't fall into action. Since testosterone levels are highest in the morning, the testicles produce most sperm cells then.

We don't know why testosterone levels peak when we wake. Most hormones fluctuate according to a daily cycle and the antidiuretic hormone is one logical example of why it peaks in the evening: so you don't need to get up in the night to go to the toilet. During our eight hours of sleep, the bladder collects a mere average of 300 millilitres of urine, whereas during the day we can easily pass 1.5 litres. If you don't go to the toilet before you go to sleep, your bladder will only really be full again in the early morning.

Our entire sleep–wake cycle, and therefore our hormone cycle, is governed by a light-sensitive hormone, melatonin. After a long-haul flight, this rhythm is disturbed and we get jetlag. Melatonin makes sure that we can adjust after a few days and that the testosterone peak takes place where it belongs: in the morning.

A great many biological processes have to do with safety and this is a possible explanation for the testosterone peak too, which also drives the libido. As explained earlier, waking up after a night's sleep is proof that you haven't been eaten or killed, and you can conclude that you are in a safe environment. You have the opportunity for a bit of sex, right at the time your libido is high and your sperm factory is in full swing.

Each testicle consists of a network of tubes. The sperm cells come off the assembly line into these tubes; in young men this can be thousands per second. With this fast production tempo it's easy to forget that it takes around 70 days to produce one sperm cell. At that point, they aren't fully mature: the tail doesn't yet move. The sperm cells first have to learn to swim. Only after maturing for two weeks in the epididymis (the structure next to the testicle that makes the connection between testicle and seminal duct) are they ready to conquer the outside world.

Both testicles do exactly the same thing, there is no difference between sperm cells from one testicle or the other. However, the left testicle hangs a bit lower.

In the Renaissance period, artists were already reflecting science in their sculptures. In 2002, a British psychologist won the (satirical) Ig Nobel Prize for Medicine after visiting countless Italian museums with a spirit level to measure what everyone had already noticed with the naked eye: that the left testicles of the sculptures were lower.

Why is that? Why aren't the testicles at the same height? What we see on the outside, is the reflection of asymmetry on the inside. Testicles are connected to blood vessels via veins and arteries, but the veins that take the blood back to the heart each have a different purpose. The vein of the right testicle connects to the inferior vena cava; the left testicular vein goes straight to the kidney, which is a lot higher up in the body. The blood needs to climb quite a bit and to stop it from flowing back, this vein has valves.

During puberty, boys have a growth spurt and their torso grows as well. This means the left testicular vein has to cover a larger distance within a short space of time and this can cause the valves to work less well. The consequence of this is that the counter-pressure of the blood becomes so great around the testicle that the veins dilate, resulting in a blue swelling in the scrotum called a varicocele. If someone gets a varicocele in their scrotum, it is usually on the left side.

A varicocele can severely impair fertility. Testicles hang outside the body precisely because a lower temperature is required for the production of sperm. The optimum temperature is 35.6°C, two degrees below the normal body temperature. This is the reason why the scrotum is in such an inconvenient place, otherwise the testicles would be safely tucked away inside the body.

What happens if you get a varicocele? The blood flows more slowly and this increases the temperature to 37°C, the testicle gets less oxygen and waste products aren't transported to the kidney. The combination of all these factors leads to infertility.

Timely treatment can prevent secondary effects. That's why children might be asked to blow on their hand during a medical examination. This generates counter-pressure in the body and a possible scrotal varicocele is easier to see.

Varicoceles are exclusively found in primates, of which the human is the most populous species. They never occur in four-legged creatures because their venous blood doesn't have to overcome gravity. While early man walked predominantly on their hands and feet, they didn't suffer from them either. The trouble began when a certain species decided to live on two feet. Varicoceles prove that evolution is not always logical: otherwise nature would have selected individuals whose left testicular vein connected to the inferior vena cava as well.

Many people have probably never thought about it, but the asymmetrical position of the testicles explains why most men's penises hang to the left in their underwear. There is a bit more room to rest their penis there.

While I was writing this book, I received a telephone call from a journalist who was writing an article about the penis hanging to the left or right. He wanted to test the claim that there is a link between the dominant side of your brain and the side where you prefer your penis to be in your underwear. The penis of right-handed men is supposed to hang to the left more often than the penis of left-handed men.

... the asymmetrical position of the testicles explains why most men's penises hang to the left

That was news to me. I'd never come across such a study in scientific literature on urology. Not surprisingly either: the author of the study turned out to be a psychologist, someone whose day-to-day work doesn't involve the urological architecture of the human body.

At the end of the 1990s, this psychologist had based his study on research carried out between 1938 and 1963. During that period, the Kinsey Institute in the United States had asked 6,500 men about their penis and whether they were left- or right-handed. It appeared that 80 per cent of right-handed men carried their penis on the left, compared with 75 per cent of left-handed men. The Canadian psychologist saw a link between the asymmetry of the brain and the position of the testicles. He also thought he saw connections with infertility and testicular cancer.

You can prove a lot with figures, but if you look critically at the original study and the later conclusions of the psychologist, the only conclusion to draw is that there is no science behind it. To start with, it involved self-reporting by subjects, which isn't the most accurate research method. To then conclude from this data that the dominance of one side of the brain determines which hand you prefer to use *and* which testicle hangs lowest is nuts. It's not science.

However, one thing is certain: most men are right-handed and the penis of most right-handed men hangs to the left. Precisely because the left testicle of most men – right- or left-handed – tends to hang a bit lower.

In the past, when trousers were still tailor-made, the tailor would ask his male customers, 'Do you dress to the left or right?' They would then make that side of the trouser leg a little bit wider for more comfort.

This question is no longer relevant because most men wear underwear. There are websites that sell underpants where your penis hangs nicely in the middle and can't, so to speak, go askew. But that's even more nonsensical than the link between right-handedness and hanging to the left.

The prostate

The prostate is like an orange. It has flesh (the prostate tissue), around which is the peel (the prostate capsule). The urethra passes through this gland.

The prostate takes its name from the Greek word *prostates,* which means 'protector' or 'guardian'. But the prostate doesn't actually protect anything. Its main function is to secrete a fluid that makes up around 20 to 30 per cent of ejaculate. The fluid is slightly alkaline, so it neutralises the acidity of the vagina and keeps the sperm alive for longer.

To work properly, the prostate needs male hormones, of which the most important is testosterone, which is produced in the testicles. So long as it works as it should, men don't really notice their prostate.

Most only become aware of it when something is wrong. Cancer is probably the first thing that comes to mind, but there is also a condition called benign prostatic hyperplasia, a non-cancerous enlargement of the prostate. The tissue swells up and compresses the urethra. The condition often runs in the family. We either treat the prostate with medication or remove the swelling with an operation. A prostate resection probably doesn't sound very nice, but it is a procedure that entails no risk of incontinence and doesn't make your penis shorter.

After a prostate resection you will ejaculate less or even no semen, because there is less prostate tissue to make the fluid. And the large part of what is produced ends up in the bladder. We call this retrograde ejaculation.

A malignant tumour – i.e. cancer – requires more drastic measures. Prostate cancer develops around the capsule – the shell or peel – and requires us to remove the entire organ. Your urethra and therefore your penis will be shorter as a result. The procedure holds risks such as incontinence and even impotence: you can't hold your urine in as well and your erection fails.

Men whose prostate has been entirely removed don't ejaculate at all any more. Your orgasm simply delivers a dry shot. That's a really big difference. Operating eliminates the hassle of sticky sperm, but it can be a real downer for your sex life psychologically.

Can you prevent prostate problems? Of course. It's good for the prostate to ejaculate regularly. As a urologist, I can recommend this to everyone.

A study involving 32,000 men – a remarkable number – showed that men who ejaculate more than 21 times a month between the age of 20 and 40, have a 20 per cent lower chance of getting prostate cancer.

The figures show a real paradox. We know that testosterone promotes prostate cancer: the higher your testosterone level, the higher the risk. This is why we chemically castrate men with metastatic prostate cancer ('metastatic' cancer is when cells break from the primary tumour to move around the body) to control the tumours. Now, you would have thought that men who manage to ejaculate more than 21 times a month have a high sex drive and therefore a high testosterone level, but it appears that the frequent ejaculations neutralise the harmful effect of testosterone on the prostate.

One reservation is that 21 ejaculations per month is an awful lot: you'd have to ejaculate on average every day and a half. Or, two days in three. This means a lot of men have a lot of catching up to do. According to a large study in Flanders, the average man has sex once a week, which totals a mere four ejaculations per month. To prevent cancer, that figure could definitely do with being higher.

According to a large study in Flanders, the average man has sex once a week, which totals a mere four ejaculations per month.

Generally speaking, you can't ejaculate too often. Ejaculating too *little* is unhealthy for the prostate. But aside from physical health there is also mental health, and that's where the problem lies in men who masturbate excessively or suffer from sex addiction.

Pre-ejaculate or precum is the slimy clear fluid that comes out of the urethra when you are sexually aroused. It is a lubricant to prepare the urethra for ejaculation and it can also act as an extra lubricant in the case of sexual contact with penetration.

The precum is produced by two small glands deep inside the urethra (Cowper's glands) and the amount can vary individually from nothing at all to annoyingly too much. An obnoxious amount of precum is exceptional and the treatment is very often frustrating for the doctor and the patient. In principle, pre-seminal fluid does not contain sperm cells, but if you ejaculate in quick succession, sperm cells from the previous ejaculation may be present, so you can get a woman pregnant with precum. Sexually transmitted diseases can also be transmitted through precum.

Ejaculation

Semen has one function: to get sperm cells to the right place in order to fertilise the egg. But first that semen must be in the right place itself. This is done by ejaculation, whereby semen leaves the penis with a reasonable amount of force to get as near as possible to the entrance of the womb.

From the outside, an ejaculation looks like a very simple process, but inside the body a very complex process is taking place. It's very lucky that we don't have to think about it, or the majority of ejaculations would be destined to fail.

So what goes on inside the male body?

The mechanism of ejaculation can be best compared to the principle of an air rifle. The pressure increases in the closed-off tube, shooting the contents of the tube outwards. The contents, the semen, come from three sources.

Let's start with the two epididymides, which consist of very fine tubes. This is where the sperm cells mature for a couple of weeks so that they can swim well. The sperm cells stay in the epididymis for two to four weeks, waiting for their moment of glory.

When an orgasm is on its way, the highway suddenly opens: the vas deferens. A milking action takes place in the testicles and the epididymides contract, and further forward milking action of the muscles in the wall of the vas deferens will make the sperm cells move forward.

With a limited amount of fluid, which along with the sperm cells only makes up 10 per cent of the ejaculate, the sperm cells move to their final filling station, the *seminal vesicles*. The two seminal vesicles (which are glands that are three centimetres in length, and lie next to and behind the prostate) are like food trucks; there the sperm cells are immersed in a solution rich in sugars, salts, minerals and proteins. This fluid makes up 70 per cent of the final semen.

To finish the mixture, the prostate also does its bit. The mildly alkaline prostatic fluid accounts for 20 per cent of the fluid that makes up the semen.

Now the mixture needs to be ejected – sperm cells can't jump out of the penis by themselves. There is an explosion of force in the muscles. The capsule around the prostate and the seminal vesicles contract, and the sperm cells are ready for lift-off.

But we're not quite there yet. For a successful ejaculation, the bladder exit needs to be closed. The bladder has two sphincter muscles, one that we can control and one that is completely autonomous. During orgasm, the automatic sphincter muscle located at the bladder exit closes so that the semen can't get into the bladder where it would dissolve in the urine. Meanwhile, the voluntary sphincter muscle located just past the prostate opens wide: the path is clear.

The mechanism of ejaculation can be best compared to the principle of an air rifle.

Now it's the turn of the pelvic floor muscles located under the urethra. At rest, the pelvic floor is like a hammock. If it hangs down well, the muscles exert more force when they contract. The pelvic floor is the catapult that gives the sperm the last push.

Everything is ready. The pelvic floor contracts. There is excess pressure in the urethra. The sperm has no choice but to shoot outwards, straight through the penis.

According to the song 'Oh La La La' by Belgian rock band TC Matic, having a small penis isn't a problem, so long as you can shoot a long way. But even the force of the ejaculation is unimportant – there is no relation to fertility. In a manner of speaking, it is enough to deliver your sperm to the front door, without actual penetration: sperm are very good swimmers.

The deeper the penis penetrates the vagina, and therefore the closer it gets to the womb, the slightly higher the chance of fertilisation; but any kind of penetration is in fact more than enough. Just like penis length, ejaculation force is a *symbol* of fertility rather than proof of fertility. Apart from the spectacle value, ejaculating a long way is of no importance. When healthy men think they don't ejaculate far enough, they are often comparing themselves with porn films. Porn isn't bad in itself, but it idealises everything. Men in porn films usually ejaculate a long way and in large quantities, but as I've said before, that isn't the norm.

Ten thousand years ago, the force of ejaculation might have been relevant. In a dangerous environment, a woman had to get to safety straight after the act and it was an advantage if you could ejaculate your sperm past the cervix.

Nowadays, men ejaculate with varying force, both in terms of ejaculations by the same man and ejaculations between different men. You can score yourself if you want: there's a scale from zero to three.

If your sperm ends up in your pubic hair while you're lying on your back, that's a score of zero. Between your **If you ejaculate past your nipples, that's a score of three.** pubic hair and navel is a score of one, between your navel and your nipples is a score of two. If you ejaculate past your nipples, that's a score of three. This scale has no significance, unless you like figures.

The sensory stimuli on your penis set ejaculation in motion, but they don't work alone. Other factors can intensify ejaculation further still. Sexual arousal is a combination of libido, fantasy, visual stimulation and pheromones, and then a few more stimuli on top during the sexual activity itself. The words or simple groan of your sexual partner may stimulate you further; some people even like a bit of pain.

A very specific stimulus comes from the vagina. When a woman climaxes, her pelvic floor contracts and the penis is squeezed. The additional pressure on the erectile tissue can be the final stimulus required to trigger ejaculation.

There are men who try to increase the sensation – with a wash basin. When they masturbate, they tap their penis against the edge of the wash basin just before climaxing. The sudden increase in pressure on the erectile tissue can give their ejaculation extra strength.

There is nothing wrong with this in itself, but I would be careful. If you tap too hard in your excitement, you could cause an injury. In the worst-case scenario, excessive scar tissue would grow, as with Peyronie's disease. Then you'd suffer from pain, get a bent erection or you might not be able to get an erection at all. If you don't want to take any risks, you can squeeze your penis firmly when you feel you are about to orgasm. This mimics the contraction of the vagina just as well.

Age also plays a role in the force of ejaculation. Generally speaking, younger men have more forceful ejaculations. That's to do with the strength of the pelvic floor – something you can practise. The pelvic floor needs to be able to move sufficiently upwards to generate force. We can take the example of the bow and arrow to illustrate this. If the bow is very bent and the arrow is pulled a long way back, this creates a lot of force – provided you have a strong bow.

If the bow is hardly bent, you can't generate enough force and the arrow swiftly falls to the ground. Boys born with bladder exstrophy (an open bladder) or open urethra often have a wide pelvis. This means the pelvic floor doesn't hang as deeply and covers less distance when it moves upwards. The pelvic floor then doesn't exert enough pressure on the urethra. These boys often have a weak ejaculation.

Some men don't ejaculate at all when they orgasm, although their testicles still produce sperm. If the automatic sphincter muscle at the bladder exit doesn't work properly, the sperm shoots in the wrong direction (retrograde ejaculation). Instead of shooting out, it heads towards the bladder when the pressure increases. Retrograde ejaculation can be caused by prostate resection or certain medications.

Suicidal soldiers

D-Day. The troops are about to land on a hostile coastline.

The male orgasm is the beginning of the battle of life and death. Everything contracts to get as much semen out as possible. If a woman orgasms too, everything contracts to get as much semen *in* as possible.

In three waves of attack, millions of sperm speed towards their first target, the vagina. One millilitre of semen contains around 20 million sperm, so that's an average troop size of one hundred million men.

The soldiers are minuscule: sperm cells hold the record for the smallest human cells. Their head measures 0.005 millimetres long and 0.003 millimetres wide. Their tail is 0.05 millimetres

If a woman isn't fertile, the sperm come up against a mucus plug in the cervix and their mission is over already.

long. Sperm use this tail to propel themselves forwards, at a speed of one to three millimetres per minute. The thicker midpiece at the base of the tail contains the mitochondria, the energy stations.

The invasion has only just begun and countless sperm fall at once. The troops have landed in an inhospitable acid bath; the acid in the vagina burns through their delicate cell wall. At the same time, the vagina moves them on: it contracts during orgasm and the increase in pressure gives the semen the necessary push to escape from the corrosive juices.

The sperm are not just abandoned to their fate: the seminal fluid contains enough ingredients to keep the gallant soldiers alive for a day or two. Fresh sperm can even fertilise an egg up to 72 hours after ejaculation.

But for this, the sperm must reach the fallopian tubes. The only way out of the acidic vagina is through the cervix, the entrance to the womb.

If a woman isn't fertile, the sperm come up against a mucus plug in the cervix and their mission is over already. If the woman is ready to be fertilised, hormones dissolve the plug. The swimmers wriggle their way through the narrow opening. It's a tough battle and it's each man for himself. Sperm that don't make it past the cervix are quickly devoured by the acidic environment of the vagina.

As soon as they have conquered the cervix and entered the uterine cavity, the survivors land on a conveyor belt. Peristalsis, the same motion that drove them out of the scrotum, drives them onwards, higher and higher up the womb, until a new barrier stands in their way: the openings to the two fallopian tubes. These openings are very narrow, only the strongest swimmers make it through. Sperm with an abnormal head or tail have virtually no chance of making it.

Those who manage to get past this obstacle can rest on the next conveyor belt. The lining of the fallopian tubes is covered with small hair-like projections (cilia), which undulate inwards, and the wall contracts in waves to move them on too.

At this point, there'll only be a hundred or so sperm left on each side. Sperm that have inadvertently made it to the wrong fallopian tube can kiss their ambitions goodbye. There is no way back, there's nothing they can do to stop the force of the conveyor belt. Bad luck: they are disqualified and swim into the abdominal cavity.

In the fallopian tube containing the egg, the final sprint begins. There can only be one winner: the sperm that reaches the egg first. If he's still got enough left in him for one final leg, he'll pass through the egg wall. As soon as a sperm is inside, the egg locks its door irreversibly. There are no podium places or honourable mentions: latecomers come up against an impenetrable wall.

Most fertilisations take place shortly after intercourse. Fast, well-launched sperm can reach the egg after fifteen minutes or so. Equally, it might take them a few days to reach their destination.

Fertilisation itself is a glorious moment, but it leaves a real battlefield behind, a grave for millions of unknown soldiers. While the egg and sperm fuse, white blood cells clean up the rear-guard who got there too late. White blood cells have no mercy, there are no prisoners of war. All survivors come to an inglorious end.

It seems absurd to slaughter so many sperm, but in the end there is one purpose: to have as great a chance as possible of strong offspring. Compare it to the Tour de France. Without killer mountain rides, almost every cyclist would be a candidate for the final victory. But you want the best man to win, so the course has to be difficult and challenging. The winner takes it all, because the rest weren't good enough.

Such a hard battle gives no certainty about a perfect outcome – who knows, maybe the best participant got unlucky and broke down en route. But life isn't about achieving perfect outcomes either, and a good job too.

False start

You're ready. The countdown begins.

Three...

Two...

And you spring out of the starting blocks. Straight away you realise: *Oh no, I set off too soon.* False start.

That's what ejaculatio praecox, or premature ejaculation, feels like.

At some point there must have been an evolutionary advantage in climaxing quickly. A long time ago, premature ejaculations probably weren't premature at all, but quite normal.

Now that sex and reproduction aren't so inextricably linked and sex has first and foremost become a pleasurable pastime, ejaculating quickly is more of a disadvantage than an advantage. Just like someone revealing the end of an exciting film halfway through.

The most visible benchmark when it comes to climaxing differs greatly from the day-to-day reality in the bedroom. In porn films, couples always climax together, with bodily fluids flying through the air. Just like giants and dragons from childhood fairytales and fantasies, the sexual antics in pornography are more than anything the imagination of the screenwriter and producer. Don't model yourself on the exaggerations of people who want to earn big dollars.

Science gives us a different picture. The average intravaginal ejaculation latency time – the time between penetrating the vagina and climaxing – is about two to three minutes. For premature ejaculators, we are sometimes talking about a mere few seconds.

A long time ago, premature ejaculations probably weren't premature at all, but quite normal.

If you are wondering how you can increase this latency time, you need to know where the problem lies: not in your penis, but in your brain. The button in the control room is pressed too quickly. Some men can even ejaculate just by *thinking* about it – these men can quite rightly be called deep penile philosophers.

If you want to do something about premature ejaculation, there are three steps to take. First, you have to understand which body parts are involved and how the overall mechanism works. This is important in order to see that you are not doing anything wrong per se.

Men who climax too soon, and have a problem with this, need to learn to recognise the moment of no going back. Before that moment they need to divert their attention, or completely forget the idea of climaxing. Think about something else – for example, the fact that your salary still hasn't been paid, but your rent could be debited from your account at any time.

A phenomenon similar to premature ejaculation is giggle incontinence. This happens mainly in young, pre-pubescent girls. If they get the giggles, they know that a time will come when they will wet their pants. They have a trick up their sleeves to prevent this: an elastic band around their wrist. By pulling it hard and snapping it against their wrist, they send a pain signal to their brain. This makes their brain think about something else.

Can this tactic work for men? It's hard to say, because unlike urinating while laughing, the urge to climax remains high during sex. It could help to pinch your skin hard, but that won't make your sex life any more enjoyable if you have to do that every time you have sex.

If a couple's sex life is suffering due to premature ejaculation, sex therapists teach the classic squeeze technique: when a man feels his ejaculation is on the way, he asks his partner to squeeze his penis hard and distract him. Unfortunately this action also resembles the contraction of the pelvic floor during a female orgasm, so it might make you climax even more quickly. From my patients, I know that some couples are perfectly attuned and they successfully interrupt the ejaculation cycle using this method. For others, it isn't quite so easy.

In the long term, it's better to learn to be more aware of your penis and its ejaculation. After all, arousal takes place in your brain and at a certain point the arousal gets so great it starts a chain reaction that can't be stopped. Before the White House in your head pushes the red button, you need to ask whether or not you can postpone the nuclear option. However, that requires a lot of concentration.

As soon as you are aware of what the underlying mechanisms are in premature ejaculation, you enter the next phase. Then you can try to control the things you can actually control. For example, you can train your pelvic floor muscles and learn to listen to your body's signals.

There is another option too: going down in the first round, scoring in the second. Begin the sexual play and don't worry about climaxing too soon. No problem. The fuse blows and your sex engine enters the refractory period. Your penis is on pause. It then takes a while before everything gets into position again. Until then, you can cuddle, caress – anything you like and whatever feels good. When the time comes for another erection, you can start the second round. This time it should take significantly longer before you ejaculate again. Men who want to try this method can take an erection pill – consider it something like a spare wheel. The erection pill makes sure the second round starts sooner.

You can also help yourself by wearing a sturdy condom or rubbing numbing ointment on your glans. If need be, you can use a combination of the two. The aim is to switch off some of the factors that trigger an orgasm. You won't feel a culmination of sensitivity in your penis any more, but you can still enjoy the visual, olfactory and tactile stimuli.

Antidepressants can also help here, too. They slow down the transmission of electrical stimuli in the brain, thus slowing down the cycle of arousal and ejaculation. However, antidepressants come with possible side effects, including erectile dysfunction and loss of libido – then all of a sudden you've got other issues to worry about instead.

Circumcision can even help slow down ejaculation. When the foreskin is removed, the surgeon usually keeps a rim of it to preserve some sensitivity. However, one Iranian group of investigators has reported good results by also removing the last band of foreskin, so that the skin of the penis shaft directly connects to the groove around the glans.

I've treated a patient that way myself. After the procedure, his intravaginal ejaculation latency time increased by a factor of six: from 10 to 60 seconds. That's a huge improvement in terms of percentage, but the man still climaxed a lot earlier than he wanted. Going from two minutes to eight minutes, now that would be an improvement.

The opposite condition also exists: men who ejaculate too slowly. Premature ejaculators might not believe it, but the other way round is no fun either. Imagine only getting off the starting blocks while the others are past the finish line. Men with this problem feel dissatisfied and their partner has long since succumbed to sleepiness, boredom, overstimulated sex organs or painful, nagging thoughts: *Am I maybe not attractive enough?*

A possible explanation is that your sensory nerves are simply too slow. Or that sex doesn't arouse you very much. Unfortunately, the whole process is largely involuntary.

Premature ejaculators might not believe it, but the other way round is no fun either.

What you can control are your pelvic floor muscles. Exercising them will give you more control over your ejaculation. Otherwise, sexual fantasies are voluntary too: if it takes too long for the feeling in your penis to reach your brain, make sure something good is already going on in there, something that enhances your sensation.

The third step when dealing with premature or late ejaculation is perhaps the most important: talk about it. Being able to talk openly is essential in a relationship. By communicating, you prevent the physical problem from becoming a conflict within your relationship that embitters both parties.

The dynamics experienced by a couple play no part in a porn film, whereas a positive sexual connection can solve an awful lot of issues in real life. For example, a woman who can pick up on signals from her partner's body can help a man get to know his body better.

Unfortunately, you do have a problem if you ejaculate in your trousers on a first date. Such people exist. They don't have a physical illness or overzealous sensory nerves, their *entire* problem is in their head. I refer these people to a sex or other kind of therapist.

Sex therapists play a big role in resolving these issues. By experimenting to find a solution, you can also introduce a form of pleasure into your sex life. Anything is possible, so long as you communicate openly and trust each other.

Shooting blanks and automatic fire

Don't worry if you notice blood in your sperm: it's nothing serious. You don't have cancer.

If your sperm is a pinkish colour or has pink threads in it but you don't feel any pain, it is probably a burst blood vessel in one of your seminal vesicles. The seminal vesicles contract multiple times during ejaculation and a very strong ejaculation can sometimes burst a vessel. It is not a dangerous condition and it will disappear by itself after ten or so ejaculations. It looks worrying, but it is nothing to worry about. Just ignore it.

If it is painful, blood in your sperm can be a sign of inflammation in the prostate or a testicle. Then you'll usually have a fever and feel unwell.

Blood in your urine is an entirely different matter. In that case, you should sound the alarm as soon as possible because you might have polyps in your bladder and they can be a sign of bladder cancer. The same applies to blood in your stools: you should immediately get checked for bowel cancer.

Some men worry about their sperm in another way: they worry that it's *too* healthy. Even if their partner is on the contraceptive pill, their sperm still manages to fertilise an egg.

There is a permanent solution for this: vasectomy. The procedure makes a man sterile without castrating him. His hormone balance, his libido, his erections and even the amount of semen he ejaculates all remain the same as before. Only there are no longer any living sperm cells in that semen. He's shooting blanks.

So how do we do that?

It's very simple: we close off the two vasa deferentia. Done. Although the testicles diligently continue producing new sperm, they no longer travel from the epididymides to the seminal vesicles. The vas deferens learns to eat the sperm cells up and then white blood cells break them down – that way no useful parts go to waste.

A vasectomy is an easy procedure, has hardly any side effects and is particularly effective, far better than all other contraceptive methods.

Now, because the vasectomy procedure sounds so simple, you might think it was just as easy to reverse. But that's not the case. We can reconnect the vasa deferentia, but once they have become efficient at clearing away sperm cells, you will stay infertile. Once learned, you can't teach a vas deferens to unlearn this trick of theirs. After a long period of detachment, your sperm are sentenced to death.

A vasectomy is an easy procedure, has hardly any side effects and is particularly effective, far better than all other contraceptive methods. The only thing is you have to be very sure that you want to be infertile for the rest of your life.

The operation won't free you from wet dreams. At some point in every man's life he will wake up ejaculating or having ejaculated. Often he'll have been in the middle of an erotic dream.

We suspect these dreams are a protective mechanism of the body. *Not* ejaculating is unhealthy, so if you don't see to it yourself to discharge your sperm supplies on a regular basis, the body will take care of it instead. See it as a workout for the whole ejaculation mechanism. Nocturnal ejaculation has nothing to do with reproduction – it's pure fitness and also prevents unused sperm from building up.

There are men who claim they don't have wet dreams and I only believe them if they are having enough sex or they are castrated. Anyone who doesn't have much sex and who doesn't deal with their excess sperm manually will inevitably find out that the body knows what to do with it.

6

The penis as a urination spout

Evolutionary chance

The penis has its length so that it can deliver as much sperm as possible to the egg. At the same time, the penis also serves as a drainage channel: urine takes the same path as the sperm, through the penis.

In a female, the urine doesn't pass through the vagina. The entrance of the vagina and exit of the urine channel are near to each other, but they aren't one and the same opening. Men, however, benefited from a double evolutionary chance – having a urethra in the penis and being able to walk on two legs means men can now urinate while standing.

The urethra ends at the tip of the penis, at the urinary meatus (urethral opening). It's not just the end of the urethra, but a special opening – like all body openings in fact. It has two lips, one of which may be slightly thicker than the other. Thickening like this isn't abnormal; sometimes there can be a cyst inside, which is rare but harmless. The urethral opening is a fascinating piece of anatomy that we still don't fully understand. It gives our urine stream some special characteristics.

Our urine doesn't simply come out in a straight line, but in a spiral. It is very difficult to explain this motion in physical terms.

Just before the exit of the urethra there is a widening in the glans. This is what gives the urine stream its spiral shape. Why is that? Well let's look at a firearm: the grooves inside the barrel of a rifle or gun are spiral-shaped – think of the 'gun barrel sequence' in James Bond films. They make the bullet spin, making it more stable and more precise when fired.

It is exactly the same principle with our urine stream. When we urinate, a strong but thin stream comes out that we can direct with precision. Without this spiralling effect, the stream wouldn't be so neat and we would splash a lot more while emptying our bladder. You see this in patients with *hypospadias*: their urethral opening isn't in the right place (it's somewhere on the underside of the shaft rather than at the top of the penis, where it should be) and so their urine stream doesn't go in the right direction and often sprays. When we operate on people with hypospadias, it's not just to correct the appearance of the penis but also the urine stream. However, we're not able to replicate the anatomy of a normal urethra exactly – with a widening on the end – so after the operation the urine stream still sprays more than with a normal penis.

If you want to empty your bladder in a urinal, you're better off choosing a model that isn't too low down.

The spiral shape also possibly makes the urine splash less when it lands – one day an interdisciplinary team of urologists and physicists might give a conclusive answer on this. Splashing urine would be pretty annoying if you peed the way you were meant to, i.e. squatting down.

What we do know is that the urine stream stays less intact when you urinate from a long distance. If you take a pee from a height while out and about in the great outdoors, you will notice that the stream divides into droplets and there is a good deal of splashing when it lands. If you pee in a squatting position or sitting on the toilet, you have a lot less bother with spray. If, for example, you want to empty your bladder in a urinal, you're better off choosing a model that isn't too low down.

Your target should be a maximum of 30 centimetres from the end of your penis.

We don't know whether the widening at the end of the urethra also has something to do with ejaculation. It seems unlikely. Ejaculation is not a continuous stream but rather a sequence of ejections of sperm. The volume of ejaculate is lower and sperm is forced out at a higher pressure than urine.

Urinating while standing

The shape and length of the penis make urinating while standing so easy we don't have to think about it. Men turn away from prying glances, undo their trousers and away they go. Only we weren't actually built for that – that wasn't the intention of evolution. You only realise this when you look at the internal plumbing of the male – or at the splashes of urine in his underwear.

Urinating while standing is an invention of modern man, in an environment where he doesn't feel threatened. Prehistoric humans would be bemused if they saw a man standing up urinating against a tree. Your penis might be protected from prying eyes, but you're not protected from enemies or predators who want to attack while your back is turned. In a squatting position, with your back to the tree and closer to the ground, you're better hidden and you can see your potential attackers coming. You don't need to look where your urine stream is going, instead you can scour your surroundings.

Our close relatives like the chimpanzee and bonobo (historically called the 'pygmy chimpanzee') still squat when they urinate and that's also the natural position for us. When you squat, your urethra hangs down in one straight line and all the urine is emptied. Standing to urinate creates a sort of siphon. Urine can stay inside the urethra and only flow out after you've finished, for example when you sit on a chair. If men suffer from dribbling, this is mainly caused by urinating while standing. Research has also shown that the pelvic floor muscles don't contract as well when you urinate while standing. That's not ideal for your bladder, because it has to use more energy to empty itself out.

If you are determined to stand, there is a trick to prevent dribbling: after urinating you can empty your urethra fully by pressing on the area between the anus and scrotum. This forces out the little bit of urine left behind.

... there is a trick to prevent dribbling: after urinating you can empty your urethra fully by pressing on the area between the anus and scrotum.

In this way, you can make the most of the handy feature that is actually a design flaw. No problems, no dribbles. As long as you are able to empty your urethra properly, not having to squat is a huge convenience, especially when you urgently need to go – it's not without good reason that women regularly complain that towns and cities don't have enough public toilets.

In Asia most men still empty their bladders in a squatting position – that remains the normal position for them. Western Europeans can't follow their good example just like that though, and for that we have another evolutionary chance to thank (or blame): the shortening of our ankle tendons. Many Asians can sit quite relaxed in a squatting position, i.e. with the soles of their feet flat on the ground. If we were to try it, we'd probably topple over. Because our tendons have shortened, we can only squat on our toes, but that's not a relaxed position. Following the Asian example takes some practice.

Fortunately, a clever mind invented the toilet. When you sit down, your pelvic floor can relax completely and you'll get less spray and less dribbling. Make things easier for yourself and sit down. You only need to stand in emergencies.

A complex system

Urinating looks deceptively simple: you hold out your penis and out flows the urine. Hey presto.

But it's not as simple as that. We might think our heart is very complex, but the organ is actually relatively simple compared to what goes on in our lower abdomen.

The heart is a type of muscle, controlled by the autonomic nervous system. The lesser pelvis has two types of muscle. The bladder, erectile tissue and intestine contain smooth muscle, which we can't voluntarily control. The pelvic floor and sphincter muscle consist of striated muscle tissue, which we can control by our own voluntary will. These two types of muscle are controlled by two nervous systems and they sometimes have to perform opposing actions.

When you want to urinate, the relaxation of the pelvic floor sets a whole carousel in motion. The voluntary sphincter muscle of the bladder has to relax, after which the bladder contracts to force out the urine. Once we have finished, the opposite happens – otherwise we'd forever be passing urine.

Another example of the complexity of the lower abdomen is this: urinating in a public urinal, with other men around you, and feeling like you need to let off wind. You try to hold it in because you don't know the others very well. You therefore want your anal sphincter to stay closed, while the sphincter of your bladder needs to stay open to let the urine out. Not all men can exercise such extensive control over their lower abdomen – so don't think the man next to you has a problem when he suddenly lets off wind in a public toilet. Urinating is way more complex than what goes on in your heart.

The complex system is likely to malfunction as we get older. The same evolutionary chance that for a long time was viewed an advantage often becomes a disadvantage. The problem is that the urethra passes through the prostate, the crossroads where the various components of semen also meet. When men get problems with their prostate, this also affects their urine flow.

In many men, the prostate grows with age, compressing the urethra. That's not good news for your bladder, because it has to overcome greater resistance. When a muscle works against resistance, it gets thicker, but for a balloon-like organ like the bladder that also means less volume inside: less urine fits inside the bladder. That's why older men often have to get up at night to go to the toilet, and they don't have the same powerful urine stream they had when they were young. They also suffer from dribbling. The narrowing of the urethra in the prostate means the urine stream loses power, increasing the chance of urine remaining behind in the urethra, particularly if you stand up.

A vulnerable channel

The urethra measures about 20 centimetres long and, because of its length, is prone to problems. It's a vulnerable channel.

Urethral stricture (or narrowing) is quite a common condition. If the cause of the narrowing isn't an enlarged prostate, there is a whole range of other causes that can damage the channel, eventually leading to narrowing. Then the whole system malfunctions.

Physical traumas and infections are one possible cause; damage can be the result of a sexually transmitted disease or a probe in the urethra. Some men stick all kinds of things down their urethra voluntarily.

In his short story *Guts*, American writer Chuck Palahniuk describes how a young boy sticks a rod of solidified candle wax down his urethra while masturbating. The wax disappears and ends up in his bladder. He ends up passing blood and needs to be operated on.

You might think, 'What nonsense, who would do that?'

But there are indeed men who do that while masturbating. I once treated a man who had stuck an iron wire down his urethra. When he took the wire out, he tore the whole of his urethra. Initially, his story was that he fell from a ladder while painting naked, catching his penis on the corner of the paint bucket. I told him that was *very bad luck* and he then told me the truth.

Women too venture into urethral masturbation. 'Doctor, I sat on my bed, there was a pen on the bed, and now it's gone,' one female patient once told me. 'I think it's somewhere in my vagina.' Our examinations revealed it was in her bladder. You can't get a pen in your bladder just by sitting on it.

People are terribly ashamed of telling the real reason. But that has to be possible within a doctor-patient relationship. We are there to help people and treat people. What we get to hear is protected by medical confidentiality, so it's better to tell the truth than make up an unlikely story. However, to prevent any future calamities I advise people never – ever! – to stick objects down their urethra. The risk of damage is far too great.

What you can do though, is check for yourself whether your urethra is narrowed. You can measure the strength of your flow using two simple household objects. The flow rate is calculated as a measure of volume over time, so what you need is a measuring jug and a stopwatch. You can then measure how many millilitres come out your body per second. A normal rate is about 12 millilitres per second, so it should take 30 seconds to empty an average bladder volume of 350 millilitres.

7

Abnormalities

Common procedures

Many men worry themselves for nothing – they ask for surgery on their penis while their penis functions perfectly well and is a normal size. Not all penises fall within the normal range though, and there are indeed men who have an abnormality. The abnormality can be congenital or acquired: you're either born with it or something goes wrong.

With congenital abnormalities something has probably gone wrong in the penis blueprint. Often genetic abnormalities aren't actually expressed, but if there is an abnormality within a family and you marry within that family, your children have a much higher risk of developing that defect. That doesn't mean a congenital abnormality is automatically the result of inbreeding; you can also just have bad luck. More people than you'd think wander around with small defects in their DNA, the genetic material carried in the 46 chromosomes of every cell.

We used to look at the chromosomes if someone had a penis abnormality; now we look at the DNA, and sometimes even the specific units we call genes.

An abnormality doesn't automatically have to result in surgery. If we operate, we do so because the level of discomfort is great or the patient is too burdened by the abnormal appearance of his penis. Sometimes uncertainty has a bigger impact on someone's sex life than the abnormality itself, and we want to avoid that.

The procedures we perform most frequently involve the foreskin, the urethra or a very curved penis. Operations because of erection problems tend to be quite rare.

We don't do penis transplants. Surgeons do transplants with hearts, lungs and livers, so why not the penis? Because complications can occur that you really wouldn't want, complications so serious that South Africa has stopped its programme for penis transplants.

Two men in the country were given a donor penis after having been circumcised with too much zeal. Both were missing a bit of their penis. One of the men developed severe herpes after the transplant. The herpes virus was lying dormant in the penis of the previous owner. Because you have to take medicines after a transplant that suppress your immune system, the virus suddenly became active. In the end, they had to remove the donor penis again.

Since then, surgeons in South Africa are no longer authorised to carry out such transplants. Rightly so, as it is ethically irresponsible to give young people immunosuppressants so early on in their life. Your immune system not only protects you from infection, but also against developing cancer.

There were also reports of a man having undergone a penis transplant in China. The operation was successful, but the man and his wife found it difficult to live with a penis when they didn't know where it had been. Although such questions are often raised in relationships, this couple had the donor organ removed again after two weeks.

Recently, the United States started a programme to help Navy servicemen who have lost their penis in the line of fire. Have no illusions: if a grenade explodes between your legs, your genitals are usually the affected party. The programme to transplant penises is planned for around 60 patients. The first procedure took place in March 2018. We don't know how the functional deployment of the new member has come on since then.

In the distant future we will probably be able to grow penises in a test tube, in line with the patient's DNA. This will mean no more rejections by the immune system and the colour of the penis won't differ too greatly from the colour of the rest of the patient's skin. However, we're by no means there yet and somehow I don't think the penis will feature at the top of the list for the most necessary organs. Livers, kidneys, hearts and lungs will be the first to find out what it feels like to be grown in a test tube.

Straight or bent?

Bent penises are common. A great many congenital abnormalities of the penis go hand in hand with a bent shape.

A bent penis isn't necessarily an abnormality. Ten to twenty per cent of men have an erect penis with a slightly upward curvature, in other words a penis that bends towards the abdomen. That is normal. More than that, it makes ease of penetration possible, particularly in the missionary position – still the most popular position for heterosexual couples.

This particular position makes humans an exception within the animal kingdom. Most mammals, including our close relatives the gorilla and chimpanzee, have sexual contact without looking at each other. Only bonobos follow the example of humans. Humans and bonobos are the only mammals with a deviating vaginal angle, so the missionary position is also the most comfortable.

It is impossible to establish whether this deviating angle is the cause of the missionary position or the consequence. However, we assume that the first hunter-gatherers had sex doggy-style and that the missionary position only appeared when humans felt safe, for example in caves or early huts.

The natural upward curvature of the penis fits perfectly with the orientation of the vagina and in this respect it's an adaptation rather than an abnormality. During intercourse, the vagina also forces a straight penis to bend, without this causing any discomfort.

The slightly bent shape of the penis is primarily due to the shape of the erectile tissue and suspensory ligament, which makes the erect penis follow the oblique edge of the pubic bone. This makes it perfectly aligned for a smooth entrance.

However, some men undergo a false penis extension, where that ligament is cut. This makes their penis look longer when flaccid, but when erect they complain of instability. Their penis doesn't stand up properly and sometimes it even points down to the ground. It is also quite loose. The result is that penetration isn't always easy and may even be impossible without a helping hand to push it in the right direction.

The natural upward curvature of the penis fits perfectly with the orientation of the vagina

I once had an Orthodox Jew as a patient whose rabbi had told him that when he got an erection he should hold his penis between his legs and point it downwards. The erection would soon pass and his sexual interest would fade away. The brave man did this and the outcome was that he tore his suspensory ligament, which meant from then on his penis always pointed down, even when erect. Because he wasn't supposed to touch his erection, and nor was his wife, he could no longer penetrate her vagina for intercourse. Luckily for him, we were able to repair the ligament.

Thanks to a slight upwards curvature you don't need to use your hands to penetrate a woman with ease, but curvatures in other directions are not by definition abnormal or problematic either. If the bottom part of the erectile tissue is less flexible than the top part, the penis may bend downwards.

Moderate bends to the left or right are often seen in relatively long penises. This is usually due to the two upper columns of erectile tissue (corpora cavernosa), which play the biggest part in an erection. If one corpus cavernosum expands less than the other, the penis will bend to the side of the shortest corpus cavernosum. Symmetrical body parts are usually never perfectly symmetrical and so the longer the penis, the greater the effect of asymmetry. A small difference will be more noticeable because the glans will be further from the imaginary midline that runs through the human body. A bend like this isn't noticeable in males with a short wide penis, even if the corpora cavernosa aren't the same length.

... so long as a bent penis doesn't hurt and doesn't interfere with intercourse, you're better off leaving it be.

A long penis might have more chance of not being straight, but it's rare for this to get in the way of satisfying sexual contact. Generally, curvatures of less than 30 degrees don't hinder good sex. On the contrary: sometimes a bend adds some spice to penetration. I once had a patient with hypospadias, a condition where the urethral opening isn't at the tip of the penis but somewhere on the underside of the shaft. The penis often points downwards, as was the case with this patient. I suggested correcting both the urethral opening and the curved shape.

His wife immediately responded with great conviction, 'Please don't do the latter!' She was right: so long as a bent penis doesn't hurt and doesn't interfere with intercourse, you're better off leaving it be. The recipient might even get some extra benefit from it.

Many congenital penile curvatures occur in combination with urethral abnormalities. One example is a very rare variant of hypospadias – epispadias – where the urethral opening is on the top side of the penis. These penises usually have a very prominent upwards curvature.

Nowadays, most abnormalities of the penis are corrected at a very young age and so we deal with the curvature straight away. It's best to correct congenital curvatures before puberty, before frequent night-time erections start to occur. The chance of a nice reconstruction failing is far greater when you put it under stress eight times a night.

The principle of this correction is simple: a curved penis has a long side and a short side. You can either make the short side longer or the long side shorter. We normally choose the second option. When you make the short side longer, you interfere with the integrity of the erectile tissue and therefore increase the risk of problems occurring with the penis hydraulics. Potential erection problems are the consequence of this. When you shorten the long side, the integrity of the erectile tissue is preserved, and you don't put the erection at risk.

When you carry out a curvature correction procedure at a young age, there is one unknown: how will the erectile tissue grow during puberty? If the curvature is the result of a foetal underdevelopment on one side of the erectile tissue, we can't rule out that something similar will happen during puberty, when the penis grows exponentially. We never know for sure how an individual case will turn out, but research shows that in most cases the penis stays straight after puberty. If things go wrong, you can always repeat the procedure.

Hung bent

You don't get a bent penis from masturbation. It's an old wives' tale that your penis will bend to the left if you masturbate primarily with your right hand. Masturbating is healthy and it doesn't harm the penis.

If your bent penis isn't the result of a birth defect, it's normally because of Peyronie's disease.

As we looked at earlier, Peyronie's disease starts with a trauma. In between the erectile tissue is connective tissue. In cross-section this looks a bit like a steel I-beam. Bleeding can occur if unexpected force is exerted on this structure. If the body corrects the bleeding too much, the area becomes calcified. You then have Peyronie's disease and your penis will bend up like a coat hook when erect, or down like an old-fashioned tap.

Men often can't even remember the trauma happening to their penis. When the trauma occurs, many patients have already started experiencing the onset of erection problems, which increases the chance of their penis ending up bent out of shape. These men also often have calcification in the tendons of their hands, which makes their fingers bend inwards.

If they don't notice the actual trauma, they will notice the severe inflammation in their penis, which usually heals with calcification. To begin with, the inflammation causes terrible pain, but over time you're left with a curvature. To correct this, we can either make the short side longer or the long side shorter – here too, shortening the long side has the lowest risk of complications.

In addition to the procedure, patients are offered a lot of self-help support to help the curvature, like a vacuum pump and injections of cortisone or other medications. Unfortunately, none of them really work. As a rule of thumb, you can usually assume that the more treatments there are for a specific condition, the greater the chance that nothing really helps.

A curvature can also form after a penile fracture – an erectile tissue tear. If the tear heals too enthusiastically, you can end up with a severe scar and therefore less extendible erectile tissue, making the penis bend.

Long penises are at greatest risk of fracture. This is because of the lever principle, where a small force on a long object has big consequences. The sexual position often plays a role.

The woman-on-top position (often named the Amazon position), where the female partner sits on the male, puts you at greatest risk of a penile fracture.

This position can create forces during intercourse that don't lie in the longitudinal axis of the penis, but which make the penis bend instead. The lateral forces can put a lot of stress on the erectile tissue, making it tear. The tear is described as a heavy shot of pain. The erection disappears instantly and then visible bruising develops. Very rarely, the erectile tissue tears in the section where the urethra passes through. In this case, blood will come out of the urethra.

Putting ice on it and hoping the bruising will go away by itself won't help. Go as quickly as possible to the hospital emergency department to have the tear stitched. A speedy surgical procedure gives the best chance of full recovery, and reduces the risk of your penis being bent for evermore.

During heavy sex, the suspensory ligament of the penis can also tear. It's unpleasant, but rare, and it can be fixed. Afterwards, your penis will be no more bent or straight than before.

A urethral opening in the wrong place

We've already had the term 'hypospadias' a few times on the previous pages. This is a condition that urologists often see in their practice.

Hypospadias is when the urethral opening isn't in the right place. The urethra, which normally has its opening at the tip of the penis, ends somewhere on the underside of the penis. It could be just under the glans or lower down the shaft, anywhere down to the scrotum.

This abnormality is probably down to various factors. By that scientists mean, 'We don't yet know the cause.' It's possible that small errors in the DNA are the cause, but hormonal disturbances can't be ruled out either.

Some suggest that evolution is the cause. In the missionary position, a lower urethral opening means you would ejaculate right into the womb. That is creative reasoning, but it's nonsense. I don't believe a word of it. Hypospadias won't increase your chance of producing offspring, if only because the penis moves to and fro in the vagina continuously during penetration and never stays exactly in the right place for firing its artillery.

What we do know is that one in a hundred males have this condition: that's a lot. Hypospadias isn't uncommon.

The woman-on-top position, where the female partner sits on the male, puts you at greatest risk of a penile fracture.

A mild form of hypospadias isn't a big problem and you can still urinate reasonably normally. If the urethral opening sits lower down the penis though, it looks bent and alters the appearance. Urine doesn't flow out in a targeted stream, but as a spray. We usually operate then.

We used to operate for everything, but nowadays we don't automatically intervene with mild defects.

You gradually realise that society is changing and is accepting the idea that we don't have to operate in every case. What is important is that we let the patient decide.

'Perhaps the boy's happy with it that way,' I sometimes hear. That's another extreme and in my opinion doesn't stand true: why would you be happy with a condition that makes urinating less comfortable? In all my years as a urologist, no-one has ever come to ask me to move their urethral opening down.

I can't say it should be one way or another. Everything is constantly changing and every situation is unique. The most important thing is to inform parents fully and let them know that *not* operating is also an option for mild forms. However, you also have to tell them that it's better to operate on hypospadias at a young age.

We can wait to operate for many things that aren't life-threatening, but hypospadias is a tricky issue in this respect: the operation has poorer results in adults than in children. The reason is night-time erections, which put the reconstruction under pressure. If you operate before a boy starts having erections, it can all heal a lot more nicely.

Penile pain

Pain is unpleasant. Particularly in a sensitive organ like the penis. And some forms of pain are far worse than simply unpleasant.

If your penis is fine when flaccid but hurts when erect, you probably have Peyronie's disease. It could have suffered a trauma you weren't aware of but there will have been a little bruising. Your body repaired the injury overzealously, resulting in a calcified scar that causes resistance when you have an erection.

If you have pain in the underside of your penis, including when flaccid, you most likely have an inflamed urethra and that is usually caused by a sexually transmitted disease.

A mild burning sensation in the urethra while you pass water can be the result of not drinking enough water – your urine becomes very concentrated and contains a lot of salt. You feel it most when you go first thing in the morning. Men with this problem should just drink more water.

Another cause of pain can be a short frenulum. The frenulum is one of the most sensitive parts of the penis and it can also tear. When we see a young man sitting in Accident and Emergency with a blood-stained towel on his crotch and a pale-looking girl next to him, we know what the deal is. The victim is often a sexual debutant with a short frenulum, but didn't know it.

One day a man came to see me who had had multiple operations on his frenulum. When he was circumcised, his frenulum was cut, which is normal in circumcision. Afterwards though, he started to get pain. He went under the knife multiple times and each operation worsened the state of his frenulum.

That's the infamous 'salami syndrome': you do one operation, then another, then another. Each operation seems no more than a small procedure, like cutting away at a salami – each cut in itself doesn't seem to make much difference, but eventually the salami disappears and the damage is done.

A very typical pain symptom is that your penis feels like its burning when you urinate.

When this man came to see me, he had already been operated on around 15 times and he asked for another operation. I said no. Not because I didn't want to help the man, but because I knew that in the best case we would preserve his pain and most likely only make things worse.

Pain you can't do anything about is the worst. Pain signals travel along a pathway to your brain and sometimes there's interference on the line, so your brain constantly receives a pain signal without an underlying cause. Perhaps there once was a cause, but the pain remains even after the underlying cause has healed.

One example would be gonorrhoea, a very infectious bacterial infection. The colloquial name for this in French is *la chaudepisse* (hot piss). A very typical pain symptom is that your penis feels like its burning when you urinate. The pain pathway can be so active that it remains long after the disease has disappeared from the body. If the pain is chronic, it's truly awful because you can't help these people. The shame that some people feel from contracting an STD can contribute to the persistence of the pain.

I know one man who had his penis removed because it caused him so much pain. However, there wasn't anything actually wrong with it. He came to see me with a specific point of pain, somewhere deep in his glans, but we couldn't find a specific cause. We performed an operation to deactivate the sensory nerve of the glans, but the pain persisted and the man ended up in a vicious circle. Because he couldn't live with the pain, there was ultimately only one way to relieve him of his suffering: amputation.

You almost wouldn't think it possible, but even after his penis was amputated the man still felt pain. This is what we call 'phantom pain'. Fortunately, it was now more bearable and could be controlled with pain killers.

Penile diseases

'Chlamydia isn't a room plant.' This is the slogan with which Sensoa, the Flemish centre of expertise for sexual health, tried to warn young people about the most common sexually transmitted diseases that easily pass from one person to another.

Getting an STD is no fun, but these diseases can also reduce your fertility in the long-term.

As with all STDs, the problem lies in the fact that you contract the disease during sexual contact and that there are therefore (at least) two of you. If you stay with your partner and both of you get treated, there's no problem. The problems start if you aren't a couple or don't stay together. If you don't have enough symptoms to make you seek treatment, you'll be a carrier of the STD and will infect other people.

Alongside chlamydia and gonorrhoea, syphilis is one of the most well-known STDs caused by bacteria. Then there are the viral STDs, including the dangerous HIV virus, as well as herpes and hepatitis B.

Some STDs, like gonorrhoea, cause severe symptoms. Urinating hurts in particular and purulent discharge comes out of the urethra. Some STDs cause ulcers, warts and blisters on your penis or scrotum.

These are generally easier to diagnose and treat – you just need to take the first step and see a doctor. Your GP will know what to do.

The best tactic, even better than getting treatment, is to avoid infection in the first place. If penetration comes calling during your sexual encounters, use a condom. It will spare you, your penis and others an awful lot of grief.

8

The disturbed relationship between man and his penis

Power and apprehension

Penile abnormalities can have far-reaching consequences – or so suggests history. Napoleon Bonaparte possibly had to go through life with a micropenis and historical sources suggest that Adolf Hitler suffered from hypospadias: his urethral opening was in the wrong place. Of course, the course of history cannot be traced back to penile abnormalities, but such abnormalities can help explain the doggedness with which some rulers tried to take over the world. Men can take on the greatest of tasks to compensate for a shortcoming.

Fortunately, most men unknowingly have a peaceful relationship with their penis. They take it in their hand a few times a day to urinate and from time to time touch it more actively during sex or masturbation. Some men worry a lot about the length or appearance of their penis, or about the hardness of their erection, but these are often only vague concerns that don't impair the lives of the owner.

Only when such a concern becomes an obsession or manifests itself as psychological misery is there a medical problem.

Fourth century philosopher Saint Augustine of Hippo wrote that the penis is the symbol of male power, his energy and virility, but at the same time it is the source of his impotence and ultimate failure. When your penis fails and leaves you in the lurch, it confronts you with your fragility and powerlessness. That doesn't make sense in itself: it's not because your penis falls outside of the norm that you are less manly. But many men believe so.

So many concerns are only in the head. For example, I have one patient who has a perfectly normal penis, but he is concerned that it is slightly bent: his erect penis curves upwards a few degrees. That happens in lots of men and it can even come in handy, because, as I described earlier, it aids ease of penetration during intercourse. Unfortunately, the problem has taken on such proportions in my patient's head that he has lost all perspective. His misshapen penis doesn't really exist; it's all in his head.

... a penis gourd (a sheath or sleeve) from Papua New Guinea does two contradictory things: it both hides the penis and draws extra attention to it.

The penis is an important organ, not just for urinating or reproducing, but also for male identity and self-confidence. A man's identity is to some extent related to his testicles and penis: a man without a penis is a woman. This is reflected in language too: someone who loses his penis and/or scrotum in an accident is 'emasculated'. Many people still believe this. Look at the character Jacky Vanmarsenille in Belgian film Bullhead (*Rundskop*): as a child his genitals are horribly mutilated, as an adult he pumps himself full of hormones, but he never manages to get over his trauma and have a normal relationship with women.

In any event, apprehension reigns when it comes to the penis – whether it's normal or abnormal. Men brag about them at the same time as hiding them away. The image of a penis gourd (a sheath or sleeve) from Papua New Guinea instantly comes to mind. The penis gourd does two contradictory things: it both hides the penis and draws extra attention to it.

For naturists, the flaccid penis is no longer a sexual object and is just another body part. That changes when it becomes hard. Walking around with an erection isn't appreciated by naturists, because this puts the emphasis back on sexual activity in an environment where the naked body has lost its purely sexual meaning.

The apprehension both men and women feel about the penis is closely linked to the taboo of sex. Because sexuality is not only a function of reproduction but also an essential part of relationships, sex falls under the sphere of intimacy. This is precisely why so much apprehension surrounds it: you don't expose yourself to acquaintances in the same way as you expose yourself to your partner. And in the same way as there is an association between sex and the emotional connection of partners, the penis itself belongs to the intimacy of a couple, particularly when erect.

There is certainly still a taboo surrounding the subject of male sexuality. Sex belongs to the intimate circle and most men would prefer it stayed there. Men don't even talk about their penises or anything related in the pub, unless they use imagery that's as grotesque as it is ridiculous. Very few will be honest enough to tell someone about their premature ejaculation and how he and his partner got over it through patience and perseverance.

If you're young, sex and your penis are completely taboo subjects in conversations with your parents. I see that too in my consultations. Older adults are more rational: if you have a problem with your genitals, you have to get it treated and to do that you'll have to reveal all. For a young boy who's not yet 12, his penis is nothing more than an urinating tool so it's no big deal. But teenagers find it extremely difficult to undo their trousers, particularly in the presence of their mother.

This is really hard for these boys. They've only just discovered that they are sexual beings. Now they find their mother and doctor fussing about the toy they want to be experimenting with. They want to be finding out how it all works and all the things they can do with it. Teenagers won't talk frankly and honestly about their penis to their parents. Were it not for the fact that it needs to be looked after for the sake of future offspring, I would see far fewer worried mothers. It is because many mothers know little about the male anatomy that they quickly think something is wrong and drag their sons to a consultation.

I once saw the mother of a Turkish boy who was convinced her son's penis was too small. He had barely started puberty. I assured her, 'You'll be a grandmother, there's nothing to worry about.' Even if there had been something wrong with his penis, this boy would never have come to me voluntarily.

Often the overriding view is, 'If there's something wrong with my penis, I'll have to keep quiet about it or the others will think I'm not a real man.' This only makes the problem bigger, until it rules your life.

Imaginary flaws

People who suffer from body dysmorphic disorder have a problem with their body perception. It is a mental health condition, where people consider a normal part of their body to be abnormal and look for a physical solution. The most well-known example is *anorexia nervosa*, where patients persistently starve themselves because they are convinced they are too fat. In some cases, the disorder is so deeply engrained that patients die from malnutrition.

Body dysmorphic disorder can, however, also focus on an organ or one of the limbs. For example, some patients may want to have their normal arm amputated because it doesn't fit with their body image. It is particularly difficult to justify an operation like that, but there have been reports of patients who found a surgeon willing to amputate their arm.

I once performed an amputation of a penis in a man who had an extremely disturbed image of this sex organ. He had been receiving psychotherapy for years to resolve his problem, but it didn't work. In the end, I amputated the man's penis at the request of two psychiatrists who were treating him. The patient was very satisfied.

I have always wondered how this man could get to this point – and I still wrestle with the question today. My primary hypothesis is that he had a complex relationship with his mother and that this relationship conflicted with the moral framework of society. His urge to have sex with his mother was so great that he preferred to have his penis amputated. This was to ensure his love for his mother was preserved without the risk of him raping her. This was also the theory suggested by the psychiatrists treating the man.

This is how I rationalised the problem, but I admit that removing a normal penis in a man who doesn't want to be a trans woman doesn't make sense to me.

Amputation is the most extreme thing that someone can do or have done to their penis. In such cases, it would seem there is no trust any more between who you are as a person and the organ that represents your uncontrolled sexual urges. In some situations, a physical separation appears to be the only solution.

There are also less extreme forms of a breach of trust between a man and his penis. As we discussed earlier, penile dysmorphic disorder is a frequent reality for urologists. Some men have such a disturbed image of their penis that their relationship or even their entire life suffers because of it.

Typical characteristics include losing all sense of reality and being totally convinced there is something wrong with their penis. Often they have the delusional idea that their penis is too short. These men look at themselves continuously in the mirror and each time receive the confirmation: yes, it's too short. To verify their image, they compare their penis with the bigger than normal examples seen in porn films, feeding their frustration and dismay. They believe their own reality, even if it isn't correct.

In 2018, the press reported on a European first in Belgium: a man who had his normal penis reduced. Men complaining that their penis is too long is extremely rare – and thus reduction surgery is too. The man didn't have an extremely long penis, but it was longer than average. More than half of men would therefore have benefited if they could have swapped their penis for his, and some would have readily done a swap there and then.

The patient was satisfied after the operation, but then he suddenly found his scrotum too big as well. This too needed reducing. And so, before you know it, you end up in the vicious circle where the same patient comes for an additional procedure every six months. Yep, the salami syndrome.

As soon as you want your normal penis to be abnormal, you need a psychotherapist or sex therapist rather than a surgeon.

Men who suffer from penile dysmorphic disorder were very often deeply hurt when they were young. A traumatising moment like that can be over in a flash but overshadow the rest of your life. A typical example is having your first sexual experience with a girl and her dryly telling you that you have a small one. Others are laughed at in the sports club because their penis is 'short', condemning them to a life of uncertainty and doubt. Child abuse can also cause a chronic disorder. Boys who experience unwanted sexual touching as a child have an increased risk of having a disturbed relationship with their genitals for the rest of their life, in the same way as sexual abuse often leads to a disturbed sexuality (and other very serious problems). In her book *A Little Life*, American author Hanya Yanagihara describes very explicitly how destructive those emotional traumas and the pain resulting from abuse can be.

As soon as you want your normal penis to be abnormal, you need a psychotherapist or sex therapist rather than a surgeon.

If you have surgery nevertheless, you can expect a whole load of misery without ever finding a solution.

A redundant attachment

Some people want rid of their penis, even though they are fully aware their penis is normal. Their problem isn't that it is too short or too long, too bent or too straight, too thin or too fat; their problem is that they have a penis at all. Some men feel completely female psychologically, whereas biologically they are of the male sex. These men have a very disturbed relationship with their sex organ.

Most trans women don't want a penis and they try to hide it at all costs. Their ultimate dream is to have it removed and replace it with a vagina. In the film *Girl*, we see how the main character Lara tucks away her genitals with tape and, at the end of the film, even performs a self-amputation with a pair of scissors.

The girl on whom the film is based didn't do that, but the scene depicts the feeling that many trans women recognise.

However, not all trans women identify themselves with the film's story or with the desire to have their penis removed. Some trans women don't change their physical sex completely and retain their penis. They may well have breasts, however, as well as facial features that have become feminised through taking hormones and undergoing possible additional surgery. These people present themselves as women to the outside world and are seen and recognised as women by others. It is this identification and acceptance that matters most to them – not so much that one body part.

Up until 2017, the law required trans women to be medically treated if they wanted to change their legal gender. That also implicitly meant that up until 2018 you had to have had your testicles surgically removed, leaving you infertile. This obligation has now been abolished. A trans woman can keep her testicles and penis and still be legally registered as a woman.

There are men who amputate their penis without even suffering from penile dysmorphic disorder or battling with gender issues. This usually happens when someone has an episode of psychosis or loses touch with reality through drugs. I know two men who chopped off their penis when they were high on cocaine and who were very sorry indeed when their psychosis subsided. I also once treated a boy with a severe autism spectrum disorder who tied an elastic band around his penis before going to sleep. In the morning he chopped his penis off and flushed it down the toilet.

A trans woman can keep her testicles and penis and still be legally registered as a woman.

Even with the best will in the world, it's impossible to understand what drives someone to do something like that. That's because you can't imagine what an episode of psychosis is like if you've never had one. Some patients with a history of delusional disorders aren't sorry to have cut off their penis – in their distorted image of reality and their body it makes sense.

As already discussed, to help men who have lost their penis, we can use phalloplasty: a surrogate penis constructed from a skin flap. That's also the standard procedure for trans men – biological women who feel like a man and who want to swap their female genitalia for male ones.

Such a phallus looks like a penis and works like a penis, but it isn't a penis. Trans men are usually very happy with the result, but they've never had a real penis and so don't have anything to compare it with. Men who have somehow lost their real penis are generally less delighted with their surrogate. Their crotch is filled again, they can present themselves as a man, but the thing between their legs will never have the same sensitivity as their original penis. The functionality isn't the same either – they are henceforth dependent on a penile implant to get hard.

Masturbation without limits

The relationship between a man and his penis can sometimes be too close, so close you could even call it disturbed.

Generally speaking, masturbation is a sign of a healthy relationship with your penis. For a long time, self-pleasuring was considered bad and pathological, which could lead to feelings of guilt and impaired sexual development. We now know that masturbation is a completely normal act and that regular ejaculation is even good for the prostate.

There are some men who never masturbate, some who masturbate now and again, others who masturbate daily, and even those who do it multiple times a day. Masturbation fits perfectly within a relationship or as part of sexual interaction between a couple. It's not a problem, it's normal.

Can it ever be too much though? Of course. Some men overdo it. In many cases, excessive masturbation is associated with excessive porn viewing to keep things ticking along. Porn isn't bad in itself, but remember: you don't become a professional cyclist by watching the Tour de France.

How do you know if you're overdoing it? If you don't have time for anything else; when masturbation and the consumption of porn become such an obsession that you start making mistakes at work; when you no longer meet your responsibilities. When your masturbation behaviour starts affecting your social life too, you can safely say that it is no longer healthy and your relationship with your penis is disturbed. You might not realise it (or want to realise it) straight away, but the problems and symptoms will accumulate.

The other extreme – not masturbating at all – is *not* evidence of a disturbed relationship with your penis. There are men who are asexual without any sexual needs at all. If they don't have a problem with it, then we shouldn't make it a problem.

Certain paraphilic disorders point to a disturbed relationship with the penis. Paraphilia denotes an abnormal sexuality where 'normal' sex isn't enough for gratification. It is often innocent, but it becomes a disorder when you yourself suffer or if you harm others.

An example of a way a paraphilic disorder can show is through a man's approach to modesty. Most men cover their genitals outside the private setting of their home: a certain level of modesty is standard (although some are less concerned about their naked bodies, for example naturists). And then you have the exceptions to the rule, those who want to show off their penis to the extreme. You could say in the case of these exhibitionists that they have a disturbed relationship with their penis. They feel a great urge to flash their penis, often when erect, and some even masturbate in public – often as a response to extreme stress.

Too much modesty can be unhealthy, but showing off your penis too enthusiastically is damaging as well, not just for yourself but for those around you. After all, no-one's sitting waiting for a man who gratifies himself in public to turn up.

Sadomasochism is a form of paraphilia as well, but this usually isn't a disorder. It becomes a disorder when you go too far, and some men really let their penis suffer. If you can only climax if you tie off your penis, stick needles in it, give yourself electric shocks, stick rods down your urethra or even give yourself burns, it's hard to claim you have a healthy relationship with your penis.

As a citizen, I salute the principles of freedom and joy, but as a doctor I want to warn against the serious damage caused by extreme interventions: men have been known to lose their penis during sadomasochistic practices.

9

Looking after your genitals

A healthy lifestyle for your penis

How do you keep your penis in good condition? The first step is the most obvious: daily hygiene. Keeping your penis clean can prevent a whole load of bother. The second step might surprise you: keep an eye on what you eat.

Normally when people change their eating habits, they are watching their weight. Or trying to avoid diabetes. Their doctor will have warned them about heart disease if they don't eat more healthily. People never think of their penis, though, as a reason to eat a more balanced and varied diet, moving away from the classic Western monoculture of red meat, saturated fat and sugar.

Men who smoke, drink too much alcohol and eat unhealthily find their penis is the first thing to take a hit. For example, they can't get an erection any more or their libido is depleted. Funnily enough they often believe something is wrong only with their penis, as though it was disconnected from the rest of their body. It's their general health that's suffering and their failing phallus is just one symptom of a bigger problem.

According to the World Health Organization, sexual health is a state of physical, emotional, mental and social well-being in relation to sexuality. Sexual health contributes greatly to a good quality of life. However, there are a lot of men – including young men – who struggle with their sexual health: they complain of erection problems or a low libido, they climax too early or not at all during sex.

Nevertheless, many sexual problems can easily be avoided. Simply following a healthy lifestyle can favourably influence your sexual well-being and therefore your mental well-being. Physical exercise and regular relaxation can help reduce stress, meaning the urological machinery – of which your penis is part – will work better.

Yoga and meditation are a treat for your penis too, particularly if you focus specifically on your lower abdomen. A relaxed pelvic floor prevents painful symptoms. And mental tranquillity keeps anxiety – the biggest enemy of the erection – at bay.

People have been striving for a healthy mind in a healthy body (*mens sana in corpore sano*) for millennia. When it comes to men, I would add that a healthy body means a healthy penis. Let's look in more detail then at the art of looking after your penis.

A hygienic penis

You don't need special soap for washing your penis: so long as it's skin-friendly and pH-neutral, that's fine. Even more important than washing your penis is rinsing it well, to make sure no soap residue is left behind.

People sometimes wonder what product to use for their pubic hair and whether they should use anything at all. Well, you wash the hair on your head with shampoo, so why wouldn't you do the same with your pubic hair? There's no difference, so use shampoo with confidence.

Pubic hair is sometimes the subject of intense debate: should you remove it or not? Each side argues that their preference is the most attractive and hygienic option. So how do you decide?

Well, let's first look at where pubic hair comes from. Humans are remarkable beings: they are the only primate to have lost their coat of hair. The only hair we've kept is on our head, under our arms and in our pubic area. Men also get facial hair in the form of a beard.

There are many theories about why *Homo sapiens* lost their body hair. Some think humans were too warm at some point during evolution, others look for an explanation in parasites, and then you have the scientists who speculate that a thick coat of hair lost its use when humans started to wear clothes. That may be true, but we still don't know why we still have hair on some areas of our body.

We suspect that head hair has an insulating effect: it protects our brain from strong heating and cooling. In principle, head hair growth isn't dependent on hormones, as is the case with underarm hair, pubic hair and beard growth. Head hair can however *fall out* under the effect of hormones; a hereditary factor also plays a strong part in baldness.

Pubic hair, underarm hair and beard hair only start to grow under the effect of the sex hormones released during puberty. We suspect the main purpose of a beard is to serve as a symbol of masculinity, like the lion's mane. Our pubic and underarm hair have a different function, because women have hair in these places too and they are usually covered up.

We think smell plays an important role here. Connected to the hair follicles of underarm and pubic hair is a special gland that produces sweat with a distinctive odour. This sweat acts like a pheromone, to lure sexual partners.

Fresh sweat doesn't smell bad in general, it can even release an arousing smell. In most people, sweat only smells unpleasant when it's been hanging around for too long in an environment full of bacteria, like under the arms. Some people get unlucky with the microbiome in this area, which makes their sweat smell bad really quickly.

Humans have to live with the fact that their sense of smell has severely degenerated. Bad odours don't disturb us as quickly, unless we are very close to the source, but nor do we experience how a bodily scent can attract us from afar. That doesn't really matter: human sexuality is based more on mutual dialogue and emotional attraction rather than purely physical stimuli like smell.

However, when it comes to intimacy, smells nevertheless play their part. When two people are physically very close to each other, smells are most definitely part of this intimacy. The best proof that smell matters is the price some people pay for a perfume. If smell didn't matter, perfume would have no value.

Before humans covered their pubic area, the pubic hair protected the delicate skin of the genitals against sunburn.

We wear perfume or men's fragrance to smell nice, whereas deodorant is first and foremost to mask bad underarm odour. It isn't intended for use on your pubic area. Deodorants not only mask body odour, they suppress sweat production. With heavy exercise or at high temperatures, sweat drips from our armpits, but that's not the case with our pubic area. This area does heat up though with sexual arousal and then our genital pheromones are released.

But outside of sexual activity, our crotch is usually hidden behind trousers, which stops any kind of smell – bad or seductive – from spreading as quickly. Pubic hair is therefore less important than it was a long time ago: you can trim it or remove it altogether without disadvantaging or harming yourself. The best option is whatever you prefer.

Before humans covered their pubic area, the pubic hair protected the delicate skin of the genitals against sunburn. Because the skin of the penis has to be sensitive, it is very thin, meaning damaging UV light hits it harder. This is why the penis is hyperpigmented: even if we don't sunbathe, it's a darker colour than the rest of our body. Melanocytes, skin cells that make us go brown, are there to protect our penis. So if you sunbathe naked, your sex organ will be the first to go brown.

What you mustn't do is shave off your pubic hair shortly before heading out to sunbathe for hours on end. Why not make use of your body's natural protection? By all means trim your pubic hair if need be, but you are committing self-harm if you suddenly expose sensitive skin that hasn't seen the light of day for months on end to the merciless rays of the sun. Even *with* pubic hair, you should cover your penis and scrotum with sun lotion. A burnt penis is no fun at all – you can forget sex – and, furthermore, you put yourself at risk of skin cancer.

The thin, soft skin of the penis and scrotum can still suffer from summer temperatures when clothed. When you sweat, the skin sticks together, putting you in some tricky situations. You know your penis or scrotum is uncomfortable in your trousers, but modesty stops you from quickly putting it all back in order. It always looks a bit strange when a man re-arranges his private parts in public; in some countries this is a more acceptable thing to do, for example in Egypt or other North African countries.

As the Earth becomes warmer, sticking genitals might be something we encounter more in the West too. If you're very embarrassed about thrusting your hand down your trousers, you can use talcum powder to stop this from happening. Put some talc in your underwear after your morning shower – your penis and scrotum will be able to move around and will thank you for it. You are quite welcome to use neutral talc, but we now know that smell is important, so you might choose one with a fragrance or fresh menthol scent.

Sustenance for your penis

You can become very unwell from something you very much need: food. Without food, you won't survive, but eating too much of the wrong food will reduce your life expectancy and quality of life. If you eat too many calories, too much sugar and too many unhealthy fats, cardiovascular disease, obesity and diabetes will be lurking around the corner. An unhealthy diet ruins your general quality of life and the quality of your sex life. Indeed, a high-calorie diet, with lots of saturated fat and refined sugar, damages the health of your penis.

During metabolism, we burn food to maintain our body temperature and supply us with energy. However, this produces harmful by-products: oxygen free radicals, which are also produced when you smoke, drink alcohol or breathe in polluted air. Free radicals damage the fine blood vessels and accelerate ageing in all kinds of tissue. Fortunately, there are substances that help stop and neutralise free radicals: antioxidants. Our body partly makes these itself but it also gets a lot of the necessary antioxidants from the food we eat.

... the less fruit and vegetables we eat and the higher our consumption of alcohol and dairy products, the greater the risk of erection problems.

Unfortunately for us, these antioxidants aren't found in the high-calorie snacks sold by fast-food stands or in the alcoholic drinks (except wine) we so enjoy. If we can't resist all the tasty things the Western food industry has to offer, we don't take in enough antioxidants and more free radicals circulate in our body than it can clean up on its own. This affects our penis too. One study carried out on 350 young men showed that the less fruit and vegetables we eat and the higher our consumption of alcohol and dairy products, the greater the risk of erection problems.

The famous Mediterranean diet is rich in antioxidants and you can complement this with the occasional cup of coffee, because coffee is a powerful antioxidant too. I personally am a fan of the rich culinary traditions you find along the coastlines of the Mediterranean Sea. I prefer to cook with olive oil and like to combine a heap of fresh vegetables with fish or grains.

Fruit and vegetables are full of flavonoids and carotenoids, which are major groups of antioxidants; however, what we are most interested in is the amino acid arginine. Arginine is semi-essential, which means in some circumstances it can't be made sufficiently by the body and so you need to get it from your food.

Arginine improves circulation, strengthens the immune system and increases the male libido. Since it has favourable cardiovascular effects, it is used in the treatment of cardiovascular disease and high blood pressure. Arginine helps the body to process sugar and fat better and allows more nitric oxide to be released in the body. And it is nitric oxide that is essential for the erection.

If you consider arginine as a three-dimensional molecule, you see that there are two variants: one that turns anti-clockwise and one that turns clockwise. It is the anti-clockwise variant, which we call L-arginine, that gives the erection wings: men who get more L-arginine from their food get better erections. It works just like the synthetic erection pills you buy, but it's cheaper and doesn't have any side effects. The study that discovered this mechanism was so important it won the 1998 Nobel Prize for Medicine.

Arginine also ensures that nutrients and oxygen reach the organs more quickly, increasing stamina and sexual performance. You therefore not only get better erections, you enjoy it for longer too. And remember: what is good for the erection is generally also good for the sperm.

So which foods contain these beneficial substances? And what is the ideal diet for a healthy penis?

Start your day with porridge and blueberries for breakfast. You can make your porridge with milk or soya milk, but it's even better for you if made with water.

Give your penis an extra power shot with a *slow juice* made from kale, apple, ginger and lime. A slow juicer presses the juice from fruit and vegetables in the same way as when we chew. Unlike smoothies, the ingredients aren't shredded and pulverised, so less oxidation takes place and more valuable substances like vitamins and minerals are left in the juice.

Between breakfast and lunch, snack on an apple or pear. For lunch, choose a 'red' meal, for example a tortilla burrito filled with beetroot, red peppers, a pinch of raw chilli, red onion, tomato, whole-grain rice and white beans. Have a cranberry drink to round off your red meal.

... a vegetarian diet is best for your penis. If you get peckish in the afternoon, snack on red grapes or a handful of nuts and, for your evening meal, go 'green'. For example, fresh spinach cooked with garlic, steamed celery, steamed broccoli, and peas. Swallow this down with a glass of red wine and finish off with a cup of green tea.

Unfortunately, I have to disappoint those of you who are omnivores or who particularly enjoy their meat: a vegetarian diet is best for your penis. But fanaticism is no good either, so as long as the basis of your diet is fruit and veg, you can add a piece of meat, fish, an egg or seafood to your meal too. The good thing is: with the best vegetarian dishes, you don't even need meat. Roasted vegetables, done in the oven or on the barbecue, are bursting with flavour and are healthy too. If you do want to eat meat, chicken and turkey are the best sources of L-arginine. Strict vegetarians should try to eat lentils, pumpkin seeds and peanuts.

The list of healthy vegetables is endless, but an easy rule of thumb is this: vibrant green and red colours are normally a sign of lots of antioxidants. It is the flavonoids that give them this depth of colour. Antioxidants are also found in fruit, herbal, green or black tea and – let's save the best news till last – dark chocolate.

Penile self-awareness

Don't worry, I'm not going to start advocating mindfulness. It's not your mind I want you to focus your attention on but your body – and more specifically, your penis. This is important for your sex life and your general well-being.

I will use the principles of mindfulness as a starting point though. Mindfulness is a method for bringing awareness to the present moment and experiencing and understanding your body. It gives you insight into who you are and how you live, so that you can steer these. This all helps you to manage stress and see threats to your well-being coming so you can prevent them.

I personally am not an extreme practitioner of mindfulness, but I do use the techniques now and again. In particular, I learned a very good trick for keeping my stress levels down during a full-on day in the operating theatre: every now and again find a peaceful spot to quietly concentrate on your breathing. You can then start your next job with a fresh mind. When I was younger, I drank litres of coffee in between procedures, and I've since learned that it doesn't make you calm.

There are loads of books and websites available on mindfulness. It sometimes looks easy, but it isn't. Mindfulness requires insight into the complexity of the body and mind. To make it easier many methods narrow mindfulness down to the awareness of your breathing, heartbeat and what you can feel on your skin.

I wonder why these exercises never concentrate on another central organ: the penis in men or the vagina in women. *Penisfulness* and *vaginafulness* would be a simple intermediate stage before reaching full-on mindfulness, and this kind of awareness is what we'll look at now.

In the story of where the penis came from, we learned that the genitalia are a reflection of human evolution. The way the penis looks and functions is largely due to the way in which humans developed as a species. Conversely, we can understand ourselves better by thinking about our penis. That's the ancient Greek principle of *gnothi seauton*. Know thyself.

Men have a great advantage over women in this respect. Because men empty their bladder via their penis, they regularly hold it in their hand. This makes it easier to think about than a woman and her vagina. However, most men don't use this opportunity. They don't pay attention to the sensation of the urine passing through their urethra and they barely think about the variations of their penis at rest, its temperature, appearance or sensitivity. Generally speaking, men are relatively unaware of their penis, even if they do hold it to urinate. All their concentration seems to go on aiming their urine stream.

Men only pay slightly more attention to it during masturbation or sex because it becomes an essential part of the experience. But that doesn't mean to say they are fully aware of what exactly they are feeling down there.

It wouldn't be a bad thing to concentrate on your penis a bit better and more often, to achieve a sort of penile awareness. Like in yoga where you are mindful of your breathing, a man should be able to direct his awareness to the balance between the inflow and outflow of blood in his flaccid penis. During arousal, you should concentrate on how your penis slowly hardens and becomes erect. The temperature of your skin increases, the scrotum contracts and wrinkles, and pre-ejaculate forms in the urethra. Your heart rate quickens and you can feel the beat in your erect penis. If you contract your pelvic floor, your penis jumps up slightly. The scrotum pulls the testicles close to the body.

Being aware of all these small sensations leads to a conscious awareness of the *point of no return*, which ultimately ends in ejaculation and orgasm, something we endearingly call 'la petite mort' or 'the little death'. Stay aware of what is happening in your body and feel how the refractory period takes hold and your penis becomes soft, like a fuse has blown. The last bit of sperm, which missed the big eruption, dribbles out of your urethra and your testicles slowly return to their normal resting position.

All these phenomena happen, but few men are aware of them when they do. However, having an awareness should help men on their way to knowing themselves better.

While you are reading this book, you can do an easy exercise. Ask yourself: where is my penis positioned at the moment in my trousers? What is it doing? Is it on the left or right side? Has the dartos muscle drawn it in or is it resting extended on my testicles? Try to answer these simple questions and you'll see it isn't as easy as all that to feel what's going on down there.

Try saying out loud what your penis is doing and then check: undo your trousers and take a look.

This is because you're probably not used to thinking about it. Try saying out loud what your penis is doing and then check: undo your trousers and take a look.

You can do this exercise any time – albeit not the actual check. It will help you improve your relationship with your penis. Ask yourself regularly how your penis is doing, whether it's comfortable and what its favourite position is.

Some penises are happy when the dartos muscle draws them in. Others feel more comfortable when they hang to the left or right, or down the middle. Do this exercise and get to know your penis at rest. Take your time and don't feel stressed. You'll see that thinking about your penis will give you a new relationship with it. You will soon view your penis like a good friend, someone you care about and on whom you can rely.

Then expand the exercise to your scrotum and testicles. Think about them too and ask how they are. If you put your thighs together, your testicles will sit just in front. They usually hang comfortably next to each other in the scrotum. If the scrotum is relaxed, it will hang down. Equally, it contracts a lot when the skin tightens, for example in the case of a sexual climax.

Knowing your scrotum is relaxed and hanging comfortably against your body and that your penis is in the most comfortable resting position can provide a deep sense of calm. When they are at peace, you are probably at peace yourself. Your genitals form a relaxed part of a relaxed whole.

Getting to know the sensitivity of your penis and scrotum is a useful exercise that can help improve your sex life. We already know the penis is a sensitive organ. The erotic sensitivity lies mainly in the glans and corona, but there's more to it than that – for example the foreskin. A study carried out by our research group showed that an intact foreskin is in fact more sensitive than the glans of a circumcised man. This evidence was gathered as our research group gave a standardised questionnaire to a group of healthy men, 20 per cent of whom were circumcised.

That's one thing. But there's more to discover still. A typical characteristic of the human body is that sensory nerves come from the left and right but they don't cross the midline. This means the left and right sensitive areas are very close to each other at the midline and the skin is particularly sensitive there. That line is often highly visible on the penis. Known as the *raphe*, it runs on the underside of the penis down to the scrotum and beyond, sometimes going right up to the anal region.

The raphe is a lot more sensitive than the skin next to it, and at the tip of the penis it becomes the frenulum. The frenulum is also particularly sexually sensitive. Exploring that sensation yourself and telling your partner about it can bring you extra pleasure during sex. You can follow the raphe up from the rear of the scrotum. Slide your finger along the line of the raphe, over your scrotum and up to the frenulum at the tip of the penis. There you will discover there's a lot to enjoy.

What many men don't know is that the prostate is also sexually sensitive. Homosexual men who have anal sex know very well where the prostate is, but most men don't dare step over the threshold of the anal sphincter, so everything beyond remains unknown territory.

The prostate might be hidden inside the body, but it isn't illogical that it should be sexually sensitive. To explain this, let's take a look at the female body. Opinions are divided about the existence of the G-spot, but there are women who vouch with great certainty that there is a specific zone in their vagina where they are ultra sensitive – so sensitive that it triggers orgasms. The idea remains that this spot is related to the foetal remnants of the prostate.

By exploring your penis when flaccid, you can discover its anatomy.

Conversely, inside the prostate there is a small structure, the utriculus prostaticus, which is possibly a remnant of what becomes the vagina in a female. In old scientific literature, this structure was called the vagina masculina: the male vagina.

The fact that every early foetus has characteristics of both sexes explains the existence of similar sexually sensitive areas, even though at first sight the male and female organs appear to differ greatly.

For many men it's a step too far, but anyone who ventures beyond the boundaries of the anal sphincter has some pleasant discoveries to make there.

If it doesn't interest you, no problem. Touching your own penis, scrotum and testicles is also a worthwhile activity. By exploring your penis when flaccid, you can discover its anatomy. Feel how the urethra runs through the corpus spongiosum on the underside of the penis. The two other erectile tissue columns, the corpora cavernosa, run along the upper side and if you have a good feel, you will notice where they are separated by a section of harder tissue. That's the connective tissue that connects the two columns.

Your testicles are easy to identify in the scrotum. A separate structure is located behind each testicle: the epididymis. Not long ago, a man approaching 30 came for a consultation. He looked as white as a sheet because he had felt a tumour in his scrotum. I immediately congratulated him: he had found his own epididymis! It appeared he had never felt this part of his body before. If only to prevent panic attacks like this, it makes sense to get to know your own body.

If you hold your testicle gently between your thumb and index finger, you will feel a soft structure all over the testicle. We ask men with an increased risk of testicular cancer to check their testicles on a regular basis. If testicular cancer is discovered early, it is far easier to treat. Testicular cancer feels like a lump or hardening in the soft structure of the testicle. These hardenings can also sometimes be felt in the epididymis, but they are nearly always benign epididymal cysts, fluid-filled growths. Sometimes you can feel a varicocele in the scrotum too. Varicoceles run along the vas deferens and nearly always occur on the left-hand side. A varicocele bulges when you exert high pressure in your abdomen, as if you were trying to lift a heavy weight. They usually don't cause any pain, but they can cause infertility.

The average genitals are sexually sensitive almost by definition, but there are nevertheless differences – sometimes big – between what each individual feels. Exploring sensitive spots and hidden treasures together with your partner can help keep your sexual relationship interesting. Teaching your partner something about yourself means he or she can surprise you just at the right time, just in the right spot.

You can discover your erogenous zones together and remember where those special places are. But you can also draw up a map of your genitals to show where the treasures can be found. Note down in the legend for this map what effect stimulation has at each spot. This way you produce a treasure map of your body. Above all, don't forget to explore lesser-known areas, such as the scrotum or the region around the anus. Adventurers can even venture beyond the anal sphincter.

Manual exploration will help you pay more attention to what you feel, letting you concentrate on your penis in a way you have never done before. But it doesn't stop there. So far we have only touched on the outer parts, yet a very important part of the urological architecture is located on the inside: the pelvic floor. By training this muscle group, you can achieve an even deeper sense of awareness of your penis, and therefore of yourself.

Training for your penis

The Chinese have known for thousands of years that the bladder is a reflection of your soul. Students under a lot of stress during exam periods notice they need to empty their bladder a lot more often. And it goes beyond the bladder too: anyone with performance anxiety will find it more difficult to get an erection.

This is down to the complexity of the urological system. It is a complex system of voluntary and involuntary muscles and different organs that have to work together. This makes it highly susceptible to dysfunction and stress.

Stress isn't only in your head, it affects your muscles too and thus your pelvic floor. The pelvic floor is a group of voluntary muscles that you can relax voluntarily and involuntarily. The entrance to the bladder is involuntary, but the sphincter – which is part of the pelvic floor – is voluntary. It isn't good to do so, but you can interrupt your urine flow that way.

Tension from stress can also affect your involuntary muscles through the action of adrenaline. When you run away from something (flight response), you don't want to let out urine, so the bladder exit closes automatically. Men under high levels of stress, for example because they have never-ending deadlines to meet, produce a lot of adrenaline. This makes their bladder exit close off to some extent and they find it harder to urinate. They develop all kinds of non-specific symptoms of pain in their lower abdomen.

The best thing you can do to avoid problems like this is exercise your pelvic floor and increase your awareness of it. When you relax your lower abdominal region and dispel stress from the area, you will also feel more relaxed in the rest of your body. Doing pelvic floor exercises will not only help you relieve stress, but you'll be subjecting this muscle group to power training, with the added bonus that your ejaculation will be more powerful, too.

Doing pelvic floor exercises will not only help you relieve stress, your ejaculation will be more powerful, too.

Before you can start, you need to know where the pelvic floor is located. The pelvic floor closes off the base of the abdominal cavity. A few channels pass through it: the urethra, the rectum and, in females, the vagina. It is a complex structure of muscles and is easily as big as a well-developed calf muscle. The pelvic floor structure is the same in men and women, only it doesn't have a vagina running through it in men, which makes it stronger and less vulnerable. Because the muscle group is voluntary, you can learn to consciously use your pelvic floor and exercise it.

People use their pelvic floor more often than they think. When you hold in urine or stools, it is the pelvic floor doing the work by contracting. Imagine urgently needing to go but the nearest toilet is a few metres away. If you were to stand still – which of course you never do because you need to get to the toilet – you would feel how your pelvic floor tenses to stop the flow of urine.

You can also do this exercise when you don't need to go. When you contract your pelvic floor, you feel your flaccid penis jump up a bit – this movement is a lot more noticeable with an erection. The other muscles in the area shouldn't contract as well when you do this. If your buttocks move too, you're not doing it correctly.

A dysfunctional pelvic floor can lead to a whole string of symptoms. When men get problems with their pelvic floor, it is usually because they are very tense, often because of stress. First and foremost, the symptoms have to do with urinating, but sexual problems can also occur and even chronic pain in the lesser pelvis.

Every day lots of men and women visit the pelvic floor clinic at Ghent University Hospital to practise pelvic floor muscle exercises. Men often come because of incontinence following prostate surgery, but there are also those who suffer from pelvic pain syndrome or shy bladder, a phobia where you can't urinate when other people are nearby. People who suffer from pelvic pain syndrome have unexplained pain in their deep lower abdomen. Their pelvic floor muscles become tightened and lactic acid contributes to the pain syndrome.

The pelvis, the region containing the bladder, colon and prostate, is teeming with neural pathways and so the sensitivity of one organ can cross over to another. For example, someone who is heavily constipated might also get symptoms in his bladder. This is why you need to learn to relax these organs.

The pelvic floor also plays a role in the stability of the lower back, together with the abdominal muscles and back muscles. These muscle groups work in a kind of chain.

After prostate surgery, the pelvic floor can become too weak, particularly if the prostate is fully removed because of a tumour. Incontinence can occur if the sphincter or nerves are damaged. Erection problems are also possible.

The pelvic floor should contract when you cough or lift heavy weights. It should fully relax when you pass stools or urinate. However, sometimes problems occur with the coordination and it makes the wrong movement at the wrong time. This can lead to incontinence, constipation and incomplete bladder emptying.

A properly functioning pelvic floor is also important for the blood to be able to circulate to the structures below. If the blood doesn't circulate well, it is more difficult for oxygenated blood to travel down and for deoxygenated blood to travel back up to the heart, resulting in a whole catalogue of symptoms as a consequence. Usually it starts with non-specific symptoms, such as an unpleasant feeling of heaviness in the lower abdomen. The patient is very aware of discomfort and pain. This requires attention. And so begins a vicious cycle that you can only stop by dealing specifically with the underlying problem. If you don't take action, you will get pain while urinating or even erection problems.

It's better to prevent these problems before they start, and you can do that with pelvic floor exercises. This will also help you become more aware of your penis and give you a more intense experience of your sexuality.

So how do you do pelvic floor exercises? Simple: you can do them lying down, sitting or standing and you can do them anywhere, whenever you have the time. You can even do them when you're waiting for a train.

The basis of good pelvic floor training is to breath in calmly and not to tense any other muscles, like the abdominal muscles or buttocks. So relax.

You should exercise the pelvic floor muscles as a whole, i.e. both the anal area and the area around the urethra. Well practised men with excellent control of their body are also able to exercise the different zones separately.

It's best to start off in a lying position. Lie down nice and relaxed on your side and bend your knees. Contract the pelvic floor muscles for one second, like when you are trying to hold in wind or urine. The anus makes a squeezing movement, the urethra appears to draw inwards. Remember: your gluteal muscles shouldn't be moving too. Relax again and try to locate where you feel the tension disappear. While you are contracting, you should feel the pelvic floor lifting your penis and scrotum slightly; then they go down again when you relax.

Once you have located where your pelvic floor is, it is important to exercise it regularly. By 'regularly' I don't mean once a week but several times a day. You should do about ten or so exercises a day.

Pelvic floor exercises not only make the muscles stronger and more stable, they can also teach you to relax. A nice relaxed state is the best starting point for contracting muscles. When you use fitness equipment or do sit-ups you always go back to a resting position before contracting the muscles again.

Once you are practised at doing pelvic floor exercises with a flaccid penis, you can do them with an erect penis.

I recommend slowly building up the exercises and gradually holding them for longer. To begin, contract your pelvic floor for a few seconds and then build it up until you can hold the contraction for ten seconds.

If you do the exercises properly and regularly, a certain tension will occur at rest, known as muscle tone. Good muscle tone is important for holding in stools and urine. The muscles will also become stronger, having a beneficial effect on the force of ejaculation. Learning to relax the muscles is also important to prevent the muscle tension from becoming too great.

Exercising your pelvic floor muscles with a flaccid penis helps increase your awareness of your penis and is highly recommended even if you don't have any problems. Once you are practised at doing pelvic floor exercises with a flaccid penis, you can do them with an erect penis. Part of the pelvic floor is located around the erectile tissue. Contracting the muscles exerts additional pressure on the erectile tissue, which can feel nice. If you do the exercise correctly you will notice your erect penis jumping up a bit.

Men who venture past the threshold of their anal sphincter can also exert additional pressure on their pelvic floor internally. You can do this alone or with a partner: it makes no difference to the pelvic floor whether this added pressure comes from your fingers, a dildo or a penis. It can be a source of extra pleasure.

Toilet tips for the pelvic floor

'Making yourself comfortable' is a euphemism that describes quite accurately how your pelvic floor should feel when you have to go to the toilet. Below are a few tips for using your pelvic floor correctly when you pass urine or stools.

You can also use them when toilet training your children. Toilet training is a crucial time because if your child learns to use their pelvic floor muscles incorrectly, it's a lot more difficult to 'unlearn' the wrong way than learn the right way in the first place. Children sometimes have to go at the most inopportune moments and what parent hasn't heard themselves say at some point or other, 'Hurry up a bit!' That's understandable, but it's better not to. Let your child urinate at their leisure, it's best for their health.

- Even grown-up men are better off sitting down to urinate. This allows the pelvic floor muscles to relax optimally.
- Sit on the toilet with a straight back and relax your shoulders and arms. Sit comfortably, not in a position that makes you tense.
- Put your feet flat on the ground and keep your knees apart. Make sure you have pulled your trousers right down.
- Relax your pelvic floor and take your time.

- Let the urine come on its own and don't force it. If you force it, you contract the muscles again and that can result in some urine being left behind.
- Don't interrupt the flow of urine.
- Do the same for passing stools. It's important to let the stools descend on their own and not to push.
- A mild push from the abdomen – and not the pelvic floor – can help when the stools have already descended sufficiently.

Daily routine for a healthy and hygienic penis

Here are some tips for a clean and healthy penis that will give you life-long pleasure:

- Wash daily with skin-friendly, pH-neutral soap. Wash thoroughly and remember to rinse all soap residue away. Clean and rinse the crown of the glans (corona), where most smegma is produced, thoroughly too.
- Wash pubic hair with shampoo and trim it regularly. Take care when trimming or shaving to prevent any injuries.
- Lead a healthy lifestyle. A penis can't be healthy if your body isn't healthy. Sport and exercise are therefore good for your penis.
- Erections are fitness for the penis and mustn't be suppressed. Regular erections give the penis an oxygen boost.
- The pelvic floor muscles support penis function. Exercising the muscles separately helps keep the penis fit.

- Smoking, in addition to anxiety, is the biggest enemy of the erection. It clogs your blood vessels and leads to softer erections.
- Alcohol takes away your inhibitions, but it also reduces penis performance.
- Drugs like cannabis, heroin and cocaine also impair erectile performance.
- Obesity is inversely proportional to penis health. In plain terms: the fatter you are, the more problems you'll have with your penis.
- Regular ejaculation is beneficial for a healthy prostate. Ejaculating too infrequently is a bigger problem than ejaculating too frequently.
- If you don't have one long-term partner, or have other sexual contacts in addition to your partner, you run a higher risk of contracting a sexually transmitted disease (STD). The condom remains the best protection against all STDs – apart from pubic lice (crabs).

Warning signs

Keep an eye on your penis. If something's the matter with it, it could be a sign of a bigger problem. What signs should you look out for and when should you see a doctor?

- Change in urinating frequency. Although most people only have a vague idea about how often they urinate a day, they immediately notice when they have to go more often, particularly if they have to get up at night or feel pain while they are urinating.
- Urinating less frequently isn't as noticeable, but it can also be a sign of a problem.
- Having to push with your abdomen (and hence letting off wind) whenever you are urinating isn't normal.

- Pain while urinating isn't normal. Feeling the urine pass through the urethra is something that people are so used to doing they don't notice it. If urinating feels different than normal, something is wrong. In extreme cases, the pain can be accompanied by an unpleasant feeling of heat. This is typical for gonorrhoea – the dreaded 'clap' or 'drip' – but it can also occur with other STDs.
- Purulent discharge (pus) from the urethra isn't normal.
- Blood coming out of the urethra and blood in the urine isn't normal.
- A significant decrease in the number of erections or hardness of erections. Not to get any erections at all any more isn't normal.
- Painful ejaculation isn't normal.
- Blood in the sperm is nearly always harmless and resolves on its own. If you notice blood in your sperm over a long period, further investigation is recommended.
- Red rash and pain in the foreskin needs investigating.
- Extreme itchiness in the pubic area, on the penis or on the foreskin can be a sign of pubic lice (crabs) and insect bites.
- Discolouration of and tears in the foreskin aren't normal.
- Pain in the frenulum or elsewhere on the penis during an erection.
- Any fast-growing skin lesion, particularly if it's got darker pigmentation or if it bleeds or itches, is a warning sign of skin cancer. Melanomas can also develop on the penis.
- Excessive smegma production under the foreskin, which smells bad despite good hygiene, is a sign of a problem.
- Any discolouration or thickening on the glans that doesn't go away or gets bigger needs further investigation.

Help, my penis has fallen asleep

Cycling can exert pressure on the internal part of your penis. The erectile tissue inside your body is about the same length as the erectile tissue outside the body; the columns of erectile tissue pass under the pubic bone. The nerves to the penis follow the same path. If the height of your saddle isn't adjusted properly, this can exert pressure on your erectile tissue as well as your nerves. Long-term, this can cause damage.

What does it feel like? You can't feel your penis any more. Just like your arm can 'fall asleep' if you lie in the wrong position in bed, your penis can fall asleep too. It becomes numb and that shouldn't happen: this means your saddle isn't at the right height and a nerve is being pinched.

The solution is simple: get off and lower your saddle. Your saddle shouldn't press into your pubic bone. You should sit on your sit bones, the bony structures located in your behind. Check your saddle is at the right angle too: the tip of the saddle shouldn't be pointing up too much; if anything, it's better for it to point downwards slightly.

False alarm

Men can sometimes get themselves into a panic about their penis, even though there is nothing actually wrong. So what is normal?

- Men can sometimes have small bumps around the base of their glans (corona), called pearly penile papules, which aren't painful. Pearly penile papules are normal.
- The glans can have a slightly bluish appearance, particularly in pre-pubescent children. That is absolutely normal; it's the same blue appearance that veins can have on other parts of the body.

- A thick blue vein on the upper side of the penis is normal. This vein can become inflamed, known as phlebitis, which people are usually familiar with in the legs. This inflammation is painful when it occurs in the penis and it causes hardness of the vein (like a hard rope). If this inflammation occurs you should see a doctor.
- White bumps can form on the penis shaft and scrotum, a bit like papules under the skin. These are cysts containing sebum, which develop in places where hairs have been. Cysts are usually harmless, but if they become very big or inflamed, they can be treated.

Afterword

I hope this book has taught you something about the penis in all its shapes, sizes and forms. I didn't want to write about the ideal penis, because the ideal penis doesn't exist.

Or should I say: yours is usually the ideal penis.

If you weren't convinced of this before you started reading this book, I hope you are now. And I hope you can enjoy your crown jewels to the full and look after them as best you can. If you are in a relationship, that's best done together.

I hope I've also been able to put those at ease whose penis is slightly less normal: whatever your penis is like, nothing stands in the way of leading a full and happy life. The biggest hindrance to a meaningful relationship is usually your own anxiety, not your penis.

I often say to the many patients who are unsure of their penis, 'If someone says they like you, but dumps you because of your penis, they didn't really like you in the first place.' I mean that.

I wish everyone a lot of pleasure with their penis, especially with the extra facts, tips and tricks you now have.

Piet Hoebeke
Ghent, January 2020

Acknowledgements

Writing this book was only possible thanks to the many patients I've treated. Their stories allowed me to test my theoretical knowledge against reality – and that usually means you have to revise the theory. It is thanks to them that I was able to tell it how it actually is in this book.

I would also like to thank the people who trained me and my many colleagues past and present – they all helped form my insights.

My colleagues Bie Stockman, Charles Van Praet, Joz Motmans and Stefaan De Henauw provided me with specific feedback for this book.

Guy Bronselaer and Rik Pinxten read the entire manuscript with a critical eye and gave me valuable feedback.

My buddy-writer Tim Van der Mensbrugghe was able to work with me to get my insights written down in a way that completely suited me and in the language I speak.

Thank you to all my colleagues and friends, and of course my husband Roberto, who, on top of the many evenings spent away working, also took my absence due to writing this book in his stride and supported me throughout.

Index